THERIOGENOLOGY

Edited by **Rita Payan Carreira**

Theriogenology
http://dx.doi.org/10.5772/65622
Edited by Rita Payan Carreira

Contributors

Veerasamy Sejian, Govindan Krishnan, M Bagath, Pragna Prathap, Aleena Joy, Archana Pr, Vidya Mk, Raghavendra Bhatta, Irani Quagio Grassiotto, Talita Sarah Mazzoni, Tamer Awad Ramadan, Malgorzata Duda, Kamil Wartalski, Gabriela Gorczyca, Zbigniew Tabarowski, Marjeta Čandek-Potokar, Martin Škrlep, Galia Zamaratskaia, Alexandre Rodrigues Silva, Nei Moreira, Alexsandra Fernandes Pereira, Gislayne Christianne Xavier Peixoto, Keilla Moreira Maia, Lívia Batista Campos, Alana Azevedo Borges, Danielly Oliveira, Fernando Araújo Abrunhosa, Jussara Moretto Martinelli Lemos, Leyland Fraser

Published by InTech

Janeza Trdine 9, 51000 Rijeka, Croatia

Publishing Process Manager Dajana Pemac
Technical Editor SPi Global
Cover InTech Design team

First published August, 2017
Printed in Croatia
Legal deposit, Croatia: National and University Library in Zagreb

Additional hard copies can be obtained from orders@intechopen.com

Theriogenology, Edited by Rita Payan Carreira
p. cm.
Print ISBN 978-953-51-3477-0
Online ISBN 978-953-51-3478-7

For EU product safety concerns:
IN TECH d.o.o., Prolaz Marije Krucifikse Kozulić 3, 51000 Rijeka, Croatia,
info@intechopen.com or visit our website at intechopen.com.

Meet the editor

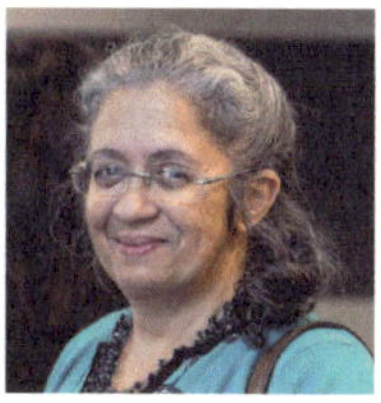

Rita Payan Carreira earned her veterinary degree from the Faculty of Veterinary Medicine in Lisbon, Portugal, in 1985. For some years, she parted her activity as a veterinary practitioner and teacher. She is now an assistant professor of Habilitation at the Universidade de Trás-os-Montes e Alto Douro, where she teaches in the Integrated Master in Veterinary Medicine (Animal Reproduction, Gynecology, and Obstetrics), in the Zootechnics Engineering Master, and also in the PhD courses in Animal Science and in Veterinary Sciences. She has participated in several joint academic activities with foreign universities. She is a researcher at Animal and Veterinary Research Centre (CECAV), in the group for Animal Health. She is currently the president of the Portuguese Society for Animal Reproduction. Her primary research areas include the molecular markers of the endometrial cycle and fertility and the embryo-maternal interaction. Related to her teaching, Rita's interests focus on the active learning strategies to develop critical thinking skills, particularly those fostering the medical decision-making and the clinical skills as well as those related to the development of interpersonal and interprofessional communication skills. Often, she supervises students preparing their master's or doctoral thesis. She is also a frequent referee for diverse journals in the area. For further information on her scientific publications, please address to http://orcid.org/0000-0001-5225-4510.

Contents

Preface

It is my pleasure to present to you a new book, titled *Theriogenology*, the contents of which include original research results and reviews flashing several distinctive aspects of theriogenology, the field that studies animal reproductive health and disease. This challenging field shows a steady growth in the past years, covering diverse aspects of reproduction in domestic and wild animals, including the assisted reproductive techniques, which have enormously enhanced the ability to rescue endangered species and provide a strong support to the high reproductive efficiency requested by livestock production.

This book intends to cover some particular topics related to the reproductive function of mammal and marine species; it is however impossible to exhaust such interesting topics in the field, as there are so many aspects still needing to be addressed. Reproductive success, as well as infertility, is the culmination of complex physiological and adaptive processes that guarantee, at the end, a species′ ability to reproduce and its survival in a challenging and ever-changing environment. Therefore, InTechOpen and I, we planned to present to you a collection of manuscripts exploring various aspects of animal theriogenology.

The chapters are organized into two main sections, one in "Mammal Theriogenology," covering both domestic and wild species, and the other in "Theriogenology of Marine Animals." Manuscripts within the first part of the book cover diverse topics, from the androgens role in the ovary differentiation to the role of melatonin in buffalo reproduction, or the available techniques to screen reproductive cycles in wild mammals, new markers of sperm freezability, and mitigation of heat stress impact in livestock, along with one focusing on the immunocastration in pigs. The second part was dedicated to reproduction in marine animals, and contains one chapter on the ovarian differentiation in marine teleostei fish, and the other describes the reproductive cycle of a thalassinidean mud shrimp species. In general the chapters are profusely illustrated and represent a great value for their readers.

I would like to thank all the authors for their contribution to this book, for jointly creating this book, by sharing with us their knowledge in the field. It was a great, challenging journey.

Furthermore, I hope you find this book a useful addition to your library in the animal reproduction field, among other many worthy books already available in theriogenology.

Rita Payan Carreira
University Trás-os-Montes e Alto Douro
Portugal

Section 1

Topics from Mammal Reproduction

Chapter 1

The Role of Androgens in Ovarian Follicular Development: From Fertility to Ovarian Cancer

Malgorzata Duda, Kamil Wartalski,
Zbigniew Tabarowski and Gabriela Gorczyca

Additional information is available at the end of the chapter

http://dx.doi.org/10.5772/intechopen.68881

Abstract

Androgens, steroid hormones produced by follicular cells, play a crucial role in the regulation of ovarian function. They affect folliculogenesis directly through androgen receptors (ARs) or indirectly through aromatization to estrogens. Androgens are thought to be primarily involved in preantral follicle growth and prevention of follicular atresia. It also seems possible that they are involved in the activation of primordial follicles. According to the World Health Organization, endocrine-disrupting chemicals (EDCs) are substances that alter hormonal signaling. EDCs comprise a wide variety of synthetic or natural chemicals arising from anthropogenic, industrial, agricultural, and domestic sources. EDCs interfere with natural regulation of the endocrine system by either mimicking or blocking the function of endogenous hormones as well as acting directly on gene expression or through epigenetic modifications. Disruptions in ovarian processes caused by EDCs may originate adverse outcomes such as anovulation, infertility, or premature ovarian failure. In this chapter, we aim to point out a possible involvement of androgen excess or deficiency in the regulation of ovarian function. We will summarize the effects of EDCs expressing anti-androgenic or androgenic activity on female physiology. Continuous exposition to even small concentration of such compounds can initiate oncogenesis within the ovary.

Keywords: androgens, androgen receptors, ovarian follicle, folliculogenesis, endocrine-disrupting chemicals

1. Introduction

The mammalian ovarian follicle guarantees two essential functions in the ovary. It synthesizes many substances, including steroids, and by this way creates a microenvironment for the proper development and maturation of a viable oocyte. Even though gonadotrophins are regarded as the main hormones regulating follicular development, sex steroids are also known to play an important role in this process. Currently, the least established follicular function is that related to androgens. Androgens were originally regarded as hormones influencing primarily the male physiology. This perception has changed as numerous investigations have demonstrated the effects of androgens such as testosterone (T) and dihydrotestosterone (DHT) on female physiology [1]. It turned out that androgens are one of the most important agents influencing folliculogenesis [2–6]. Androgens are known to exert pro-apoptotic effects [7, 8] but are also indispensable in normal folliculogenesis for both androgen receptor-mediated responses and as substrates for estrogen synthesis [9]. Androgenic actions play a role mainly in early follicular growth, whereas estrogenic roles are more important at later follicle development stages [1, 9]. The high number of androgen receptors (ARs) that characterize granulosa cells (GCs) in preantral follicles declines during antral differentiation at the same time as expression of mRNA for P450 aromatase (P450arom) and estrogen synthesis increase [10–13].

Recently, a growing concern aroused about the potential for environmental endocrine-disrupting chemicals (EDCs) to alter sexual differentiation. EDCs are one of the factors that can induce unfavorable changes taking place in the ovary [14, 15]. They originate as a result of human industrial activities, enter the natural environment, and then disturb hormonal regulation (e.g., through blocking steroid hormone receptors) [16]. Such a mechanism of action negatively influences many processes taking place in the reproductive tract of a female [17, 18]. In extreme cases, this may lead to the elimination of many populations from their natural habitats, by premature cessation of ovarian function, among other putative mechanisms. The image of muscular bodies as the model for an ideal, which is frequently carried in mass communication media, has led to an increase in the number of enthusiasts for androgenic anabolic steroid (AAS) use. AAS is a group of synthetic compounds that originate from testosterone and its esterified or alkalinized derivatives belonging to EDCs. The association between AAS use and cancer that has been described in the literature and may be related to the genotoxic potential has already been shown in several studies [19, 20]. *In vitro* toxicological models are widely used to assess the effects of endogenous androgens and EDCs on ovarian function, to understand their role in the initiation/progression of ovarian cancers.

In this chapter, we intend to point out a possible impact of androgen excess or deficiency on the regulation of ovarian function as well as following EDC action with antiandrogenic (e.g., vinclozolin, linuron) or androgenic (e.g., anabolic steroids: testosterone propionate, boldione) activity due to the fact that continuous exposition to even small concentration of such compounds can initiate oncogenesis within the ovary. Following our previous results obtained using an in vitro animal model generated for studying androgen deficiency, we have found that the exposure of porcine follicles to an environmental antiandrogen—vinclozolin—caused deleterious effects at antrum formation stage that may negatively influence the reproductive function in mammals.

2. Androgen receptor structure and mechanism of action

Like all steroid hormones, androgens affect target cells by binding to and activating specialized receptors. The types of receptors that are involved in the signal transduction decide on its mechanism of action. A genomic response is usually induced by receptors localized in the cytoplasm/nucleus. Additionally, androgens can also exert their effects by interacting with receptors located on the cell membrane to perform rapid, non-genomic actions. It is well known that the cross talk between non-genomic and genomic signaling pathways is crucial for proper ovarian function [21].

The ARs, encoded by a gene composed of eight exons located on the X chromosome, are proteins with approximately 919 amino acids. The exact length of ARs is variable due to the existence of two diverse polyglutamine and polyglycine stretches in the N-terminal region of the protein [22]. This AR region modulates its transactivation [23, 24] and, hence, its functionality. The ARs, which belong to the nuclear receptor superfamily, are characterized by a modular structure consisting of four functional domains: C-terminal domain responsible for ligand binding (LBD), a highly conserved DNA-binding domain (DBD) with centrally located zinc fingers, a hinge region, and N-terminal domain (NTD) (**Figure 1**) [25, 26]. The C-terminal domain of ARs is encoded by exons 4–8. Within itself, besides LBD, C-terminal domain also contains transcriptional activation function 2 (AF2) co-regulator binding interface [27, 28]. In the most conserved region of ARs—DNA-binding domain—two zinc fingers encoded by exon 2 and exon 3, respectively, are located. The first zinc finger determines the specificity of DNA recognition, which makes contact with major groove residues in an androgen-response element (ARE) half-site. The second zinc finger is a dimerization interface that mediates binding with a neighboring AR molecule engaged with an adjacent ARE half-site [29]. The short flexible hinge region, encoded by exon 4, regulates DNA binding, nuclear translocation, and transactivation of the ARs [30]. The N-terminal domain, encoded by AR exon 1, is relatively long and poorly conserved. It displays the most sequence variability by, as mentioned above, virtue of polymorphic (CAG)n and (GGN)n repeat units encoding polyglutamine and polyglycine tracts, respectively [31–33]. This domain contains also the AF1, which harbors two transactivation regions, transcriptional activation unit-1 (TAU-1), and transcriptional activation unit-5 (TAU-5). The N-terminal domain is essential for AR activation [34] and, because it contains many sites for Ser/Thr phosphorylation, may be involved in mediating cross talk with other signaling pathways leading to the modulation of AF1 activity and interaction with co-regulators [35].

In the absence of androgens, unliganded ARs remain in the cytoplasm. To maintain the unbounded AR protein in a stable and inactive configuration, the molecular chaperone complex, including Hsp90 and high-molecular-weight immunophilins, is needed. Androgens like other steroids can freely diffuse across the plasma membrane and bind to the LBD region that induces conformational changes, including the Hsp90 dissociation from ARs. Followed by these transformation, ARs undergo dimerization, phosphorylation, and translocation to the nucleus, which is mediated by the nuclear localization signal (NLS) in the hinge region. The dimer binds to the androgen response elements (AREs) located in the promoter of the target gene and leads to the recruitment of co-regulators, either coactivators or corepressors such as steroid receptor coactivator 1 (SRC1) and transcriptional intermediary factor 2 (TIF2), leading to transcription of genes that are involved in many cellular activities, from proliferation to programmed cell death [36]. In some cases, for example, in the low androgen concentration, the ligand-independent signaling pathway may occur. This process involves MAPK/ERK pathway and depends on growth factor

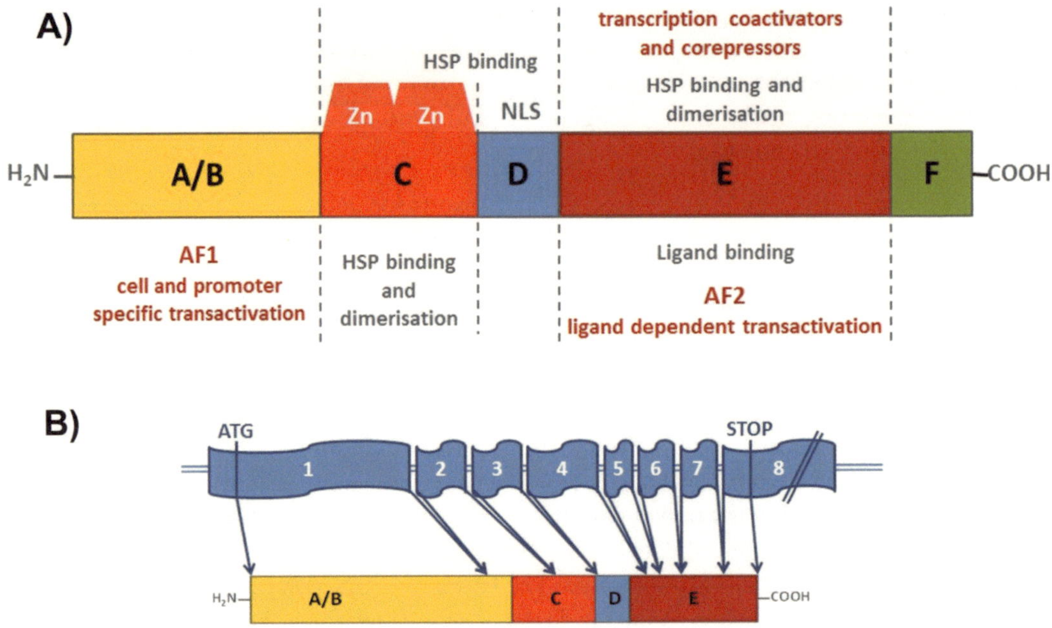

Figure 1. Schematic representation of the structural and functional domains of AR protein (**A**) and the coding of exons 1–8 in relation to each functional domain of human AR gene (**B**). AF, transcriptional activation function; NLS, nuclear localization signal; HSP, heat shock protein.

receptors. As a result, transcriptional activity enhancement, through direct phosphorylation of steroid receptors, is observed [37]. The androgen signaling pathways depicted above are collectively known as "genomic pathway" (**Figure 2**) [38].

Apart from the direct or indirect genomic effects, androgens may also operate in cells by the "non-genomic pathway," stimulating rapid effects in signal transduction through the production of second messengers, ion channel transport, and protein kinase cascades. This kind of activity involves receptors localized in the plasma membrane or in "lipid rafts" [39]. Rapid non-genomic action of androgens might be mediated by binding to transmembrane receptors unrelated to nuclear hormone receptors (usually G-protein-coupled receptor (GPCR)) that was well documented in different tissues [40, 41]. Among GPCRs, there are GPRC6A and ZIP9 that have been pharmacologically well characterized [42, 43]. Additionally, androgens can induce activation of the Src/Ras/Raf/MAPK/ERK1/ERK2 pathway in the cytoplasm, independently of receptor-DNA interactions (**Figure 2**) [44, 45]. It was shown that in luteinized human GCs androgens caused rapid, non-genomic-dependent rise in cytosolic calcium, involving voltage-dependent calcium channels in the plasma membrane and phospholipase C [46, 47].

Androgen action might be disturbed by alternative splicing [48]. This is a common event described in the structural molecular biology of AR genes. Alternative splicing is a process by which multiple different mRNAs and downstream proteins can be generated from one gene through the inclusion or exclusion of specific exons [49]. This process might occur in

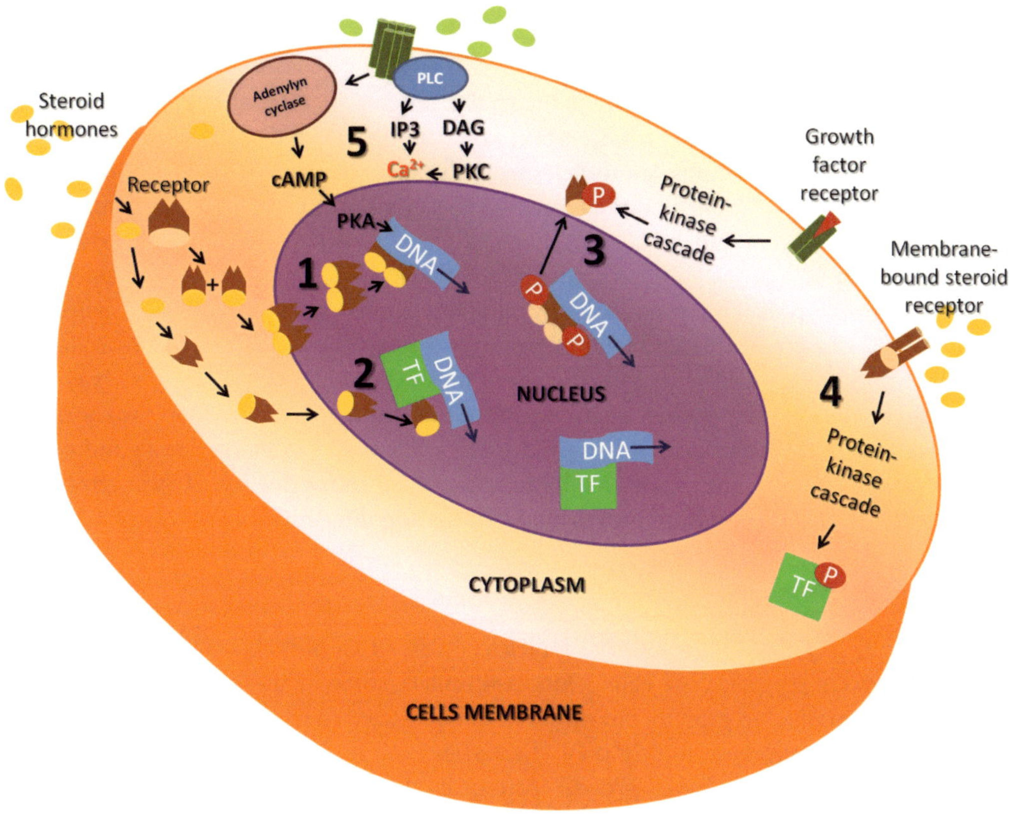

Figure 2. Molecular mechanism of the AR action. After entering into the cell, ARs bind to their specific receptors located in the cytoplasm; the ligand-receptor complexes are then translocated to the nucleus. After that, they bind to DNA as dimmers modulating gene expression (**1**). Alternatively, the ligand-receptor complexes in the nucleus interact with transcription factors, which in turn bind to their responsive elements on the DNA to regulate gene expression (**2**). Hormone-independent mechanism involves AR phosphorylation and activation, which is triggered by protein kinase cascade in response to growth factors binding to their receptors located on the cell membrane. Phosphorylated ARs enter the nucleus and bind to DNA, regulating gene expression (**3**). Androgens may also be directly bounded by cell membrane receptors, triggering the activation of protein kinase cascades. Thereafter, phosphorylated transcription factors bind to their own response elements in the genome, thereby controlling gene expression (**4**). Androgen action might be either mediated by intracellular secondary messengers produced in response to the activation of G-protein-coupled receptors (**5**). TF, transcription factor; cAMP, cyclic AMP; PKA, protein kinase A; PLC, phospholipase C; IP_3, inositol 1,4,5-trisphosphate; DAG, diacylglycerol; PKC, protein kinase C.

95% of all multi-exonic genes and provides a significant advantage in evolution by increasing proteomic diversity [50]. Although deregulation of this process may lead to inappropriate spliced mRNA, impaired proteins and eventually to diseases such as cancers [51, 52] or endocrine system dysfunction [53]. More recently, two AR splice variants expressed in GCs from patients with polycystic ovary syndrome (PCOS), which is one of the most common causes of female infertility, have been identified [54]. The altered AR splicing patterns are strongly associated with hyperandrogenism and abnormal folliculogenesis in PCOS [55]. It seems possible that AR alternative splicing may be an important pathogenic mechanism in human infertility.

3. Androgens and follicular development

In the ovary of a mature mammalian female, the process of folliculogenesis proceeds all the time, which manifests in cell proliferation and differentiation. Such a process, involving growth and development of ovarian follicles from the stage of primordial to the preovulatory ones, is a substantially complicated phenomenon requiring multidirectional regulation. From the initial pool of ovarian follicles starting to grow, the preovulatory stage is reached by only a few. More than 99% of the follicles undergo atresia at various stages of development. The transition from the preantral to an early antral stage is most susceptible to this process. All primordial follicles present during fetal life constitute a reserve that cannot increase later on, during the postnatal period. Therefore, the very first stages of folliculogenesis, such as formation of primordial follicles, their recruitment from the resting pool, and then transformation into primary ones, are critical for the reproductive cycle of a vertebrate female animal [56]. Improper coordination of the primordial follicle formation and activation of their growth may disturb folliculogenesis in mature individuals originating infertility.

3.1. Origin of primordial follicles

In the developing ovary, the primordial follicles consist of an oocyte surrounded by a single layer of squamous pregranulosa cells. Once assembled, some of the primordial follicles are immediately stimulated to growth, but most remain quiescent until selected follicles are gradually recruited into a growing follicle pool, throughout the reproductive life [57]. The recruitment of primordial follicles into a growth (primordial-to-primary follicle transition) involves a change in the shape of the granulosa cells from squamous to cuboidal and the initiation of oocyte growth. The primordial-to-primary follicle transition is an irreversible process. The early stages of folliculogenesis are believed to be gonadotropin independent. All events related to early follicular development are mostly regulated by paracrine growth factors originating from the growing oocyte itself and from the somatic cells that surround it [58, 59] and also by ovarian steroid hormones (i.e., progesterone, androgens, and estrogens) [6]. Interestingly, during initiation of primordial follicle growth, a fundamental role for androgens has been shown. In mouse, bovine and primate ovaries T and DHT [3, 60, 61] are responsible for the stimulation of this process, while in sheep DHEA plays the main role [62]. The initiation of primordial follicle growth might be mediated through paracrine stimulation, by upregulation of IGF-1 and/or its receptor [63]. On the other hand, it seems possible that androgens, acting through ARs, regulate the early stages of follicular development. Fowler et al. [61] reported that in human fetal ovaries pregranulosa cells express ARs, and the oocytes of the primordial follicles are able to synthesize androgens. Taken together, androgens might stimulate the primordial-to-primary follicle transition but still an open-ended question is that how they exactly influence primordial follicle recruitment and whether this is a primary or secondary response [64].

3.2. Antral follicle formation

Studies indicating AR expression in the different compartments of follicles throughout most stages of folliculogenesis allowed us to assume that androgens regulate follicular development [9].

Although AR expression pattern differs between follicular cell types, it has been observed that AR number declines together with follicle maturation to the preovulatory stage [65]. AR-mediated actions might be important in the antrum formation during follicular development. Mouse preantral follicles cultured in vitro in the presence of an AR antagonist, bicalutamide, showed significantly suppressed growth and antral cavity formation. At the same time, supplementation of culture medium with DHT restored the follicular growth and antral development in follicles cultured without FSH addition [66]. Similar situation was observed after different androgens (incl. T, DHT, or DHEA) in addition to in vitro culture system of mouse preantral follicles. They undergone rapid granulosa cell proliferation and amplified responsiveness to FSH [67]. Moreover, supplementation of culture media with estrogens, with or without fadrozole (an aromatase inhibitor), had no effect on follicular development, while the addition of an AR antagonist, flutamide, suppressed follicular growth. These studies allow to state that these androgen stimulatory effects on antrum formation and follicular growth are mediated directly through ARs and are not induced by T aromatization to estrogens [3]. Our recent research was conducted to determine whether experimentally induced androgen deficiency during in vitro culture of porcine ovarian cortical slices affects preantral follicular development. Cultured preantral follicles were supplemented with testosterone, nonsteroidal antiandrogen, 2-hydroxyflutamide, and a dicarboximide fungicide, separately or in combination with androgen. 2-Hydoxyflutamide is a pharmaceutical compound, which is regarded as a model antiandrogen in experimental studies. It promotes AR translocation to the nucleus and DNA binding but nevertheless fails to initiate transcription, inhibiting the AR signaling pathway [68]. We demonstrated the deleterious effects of androgen deficiency at antrum formation stage, what confirms androgen involvement in porcine early follicular development [69]. In summary, it was clearly shown that androgens enhance ovarian follicle growth, from preantral to antral stage. The main findings regarding the direct action of androgens on the in vivo and in vitro control of follicular development in mammals are based on the transcriptional actions of ARs in follicular cells.

3.3. Preovulatory follicular development

During antrum formation GCs separate into cumulus GCs and mural GCs, which line the follicle wall. These two subpopulations of GCs gain different morphological and functional properties during further follicle development [70]. The mural granulosa cells are characterized by high levels of steroidogenic enzyme activity, which converts androgens to estrogens, while the cumulus cells (CCs) are engaged in supporting oocyte growth and maturation. Just before ovulation, CCs acquire steroidogenic abilities and start to produce primarily progesterone [71]. The role of ARs in the female was elucidated by the studies of various global and tissue-specific AR knockout (ARKO) mouse models [72]. Granulosa cell-specific ARKO (GCARKO) mouse models have demonstrated that granulosa cells are an important site for androgen action and strongly suggested that the AR in these cells is an important regulator of androgen-mediated follicular growth and development. On the other hand, AR inactivation in the oocyte, as shown in the OoARKO female mouse model, appears to have no major overall effect on female fertility [73]. Using female mice lacking functional ARs (AR−/α), Hu et al. [74] demonstrated impaired expression of ovulatory genes, defective morphology of the preovulatory cumulus oophorus cells, and markedly reduced fertility. However, there are contradictory reports concerning androgen effects on oocyte maturation and embryonic development. While some authors found androgens exerting inhibitory effects on these processes in different species [75, 76], others have shown that T increases the cleavage rate of fertilized rat oocytes and that dihydrotestosterone improves the fertilizability of mouse oocytes [77, 78]. Optimal androgen levels appear to be of real importance in the maintenance of proper preovulatory follicular development ensuring normal ovulatory function. Administration of T or DHT did not increase preovulatory follicle numbers in primate ovaries [12]. Yet, in pigs, treatment with T or DHT during the late follicular phase increased the number of preovulatory follicles and corpora lutea [79]. In mice, DHT at a low dose [80] improved the ovulatory response to superovulation. Likewise, in vivo treatment of rats with a steroidal AR blocker (cyproterone acetate) leads to a decrease in the number of new corpora lutea, indicating an inhibition of ovulation [81]. To sum up, these findings indicate that androgens indeed play a role at the preovulatory stage of follicle life cycle. Moreover, the coordination of oocyte maturation and ovulation is reactive to the androgenic environment. Therefore, a balance of androgen positive and negative actions is required for optimal ovarian functioning. Some contradictory findings on the role played by androgens in this period of follicle development stress the need for further research aimed at elucidating the background of these processes.

4. Antiandrogenic and androgenic EDC action within the ovary

In the light of a dramatic increase of evidences demonstrating the harmful effects of EDCs present in the environment, it is crucial for further research on the female reproductive potency to understand the mechanisms of their action within ovaries. Among EDCs there is a large group of chemicals exerting antiandrogenic effects and blocking endogenous androgen action. We can find there pharmaceuticals (e.g. 2-hydroxyflutamide, ketoconazole) as well as environmental contaminants: pesticides (e.g. vinclozolin, linuron) or synthetic androgens such as testosterone propionate or boldione, which are widely used anabolic steroids [82]. During our previous experiments concerning the involvement of androgen in ovarian follicular development and atresia, we generated an in vitro toxicological model for studying androgen deficiency. Using 2-hydroxyflutamide, which is a nonsteroidal antiandrogen acting at the AR level, we induced distortions of androgen action in the ovary that in consequence reduced porcine GC viability and proliferation [83].

Vinclozolin, a commonly used dicarboximide fungicide, is registered in the USA and Europe to prevent decay of fruits and vegetables. It was shown that vinclozolin possesses an antiandrogenic activity in mammals and fish [84–86]. Two major ring-opened metabolites of vinclozolin (butenoic acid M1 and enanilide M2) have been detected in rodent fluids and tissue extracts following in vivo exposure that might have negative consequences for human health [87–89]. Exposure to vinclozolin during gonadal sex determination period in mice promotes a transgenerational increase in pregnancy abnormalities and female adult onset malformation in the reproductive organs [90, 91]. Our previous studies showed that vinclozolin at an environmentally relevant concentration might contribute to the amplification and propagation of apoptotic cell death in the granulosa layer, leading to the rapid removal of atretic follicles in porcine ovary [92, 93]. Besides, it seems possible that vinclozolin activates non-genomic signaling pathways directly modifying the AR action. Another widely used pesticide with antiandrogenic activity is linuron. In vitro studies in mammals demonstrated that linuron competitively inhibits the binding of androgens to the ARs [94] and acts as a weak AR antagonist in transcriptional activation assays [95]. Additionally, prenatal in vivo exposure to high doses of linuron caused reduced testosterone production, altered expression patterns in gene involved in tissue morphogenesis, and morphological disruptions to androgen-organized tissues [96–98]. It is currently hypothesized that antiandrogenic pesticides such as vinclozolin or linuron act through a mixed mode of action including both AR antagonism and reduced testosterone production.

The European Community banned the use of anabolics in Europe by means of laws 96/22/EC and 96/23/EC. Despite these regulations, in many countries, exogenous sex hormones are widely and illegally used in livestock for anabolic purposes during the last 2 months of the fattening period. Such deliberate action raised ovarian cancer incidence in both adult and young animals [99]. Literature search reveals a positive correlation between steroid hormone abuse and cancer incidence [100]. Sex hormones and gonadotropins are responsible for the regulation of granulosa cell proliferation and their physiological changes with maturation [101]. They stimulate cell growth, even in mutated cells, and this is why they are considered cocarcinogens. Thanks to their ability to stimulate mitosis, thus increasing the number of cell divisions, steroids also increase the risk of mutations [102]. Generally, some mutations can be corrected by cellular DNA repair mechanisms, but since these processes require prolonged times, it is believed that faster cell division increases the risk of mutations that can be transferred to daughter cells. Consequently, these hormones may act not only as cocarcinogens but also as true carcinogens, being able to provoke an increased risk for mutation in their target cells. They also stimulate the divisions of the mutated cells [103]. An increased proliferation rate observed in many cell lines indicates that sex steroid hormones act as growth factors and activate respective signaling pathways [104]. Although this is not a uniform view, it seems that sex steroids interfere with mechanisms controlling apoptotic cell death. Regarding androgens, in some experiments, they have been shown to promote granulosa cell apoptosis [105], while other authors have affirmed that they preserved granulosa cells and follicles from undergoing programmed cell death [106]. Today, there is more than 100 varieties of AAS that have been developed, with only a few approved for human or veterinary use. They are used not only by athletic competitors and sportsmen but also by people wanting to alter their physical appearance usually based on the widespread belief that strong, muscled body is the model for the ideal. Some anabolic substances, i.e., testosterone propionate, boldione, or nandrolone, are openly available on the Internet for use by body builders. The International Agency for Research on Cancer classifies them as probable human carcinogens, with a carcinogenicity index higher than that of other androgens such as stanozolol, clostebol, and testosterone [107]. Recently, several models of primary granulosa cell cultures, originating from different animal species, have been devised and are being used to test the effects of EDCs (including anabolic steroids) on cell proliferation, steroidogenesis, and neoplastic transformation [108]. Moreover, after in vivo exposure of an animal to testosterone propionate, an increase in primary follicle number together with a decrease in those with antrum was observed, leading to the higher proportion of atretic follicles and the lack of corpora lutea within the ovaries [109]. Following these considerations, it should be useful to evaluate the possible involvement of anabolics in the follicular cell transformation being this the first step of carcinogenesis. It might be also possible, in view of the way in which steroids and their derivate act in the mammalian ovary, to check if anabolics trigger follicular cell apoptosis, thereby causing PCOS.

5. Conclusions

In the last decades, it was proven that environmental chemical compounds exert toxic and genotoxic effects and thus form a serious threat to mammalian reproduction. However, the impact of anabolics on ovarian function has been less realized and studied. Recognition and evaluation of risk associated with the AAS use are of the utmost importance for human health. Harmful effects of compounds with antiandrogenic activities acting during folliculogenesis have been shown to affect oocyte survival and follicle growth, as well as steroidogenesis. Better understanding of the mechanisms underlying the consequences of the EDC exposure is required to implement a risk reduction measures to the health of living organisms and, more generally, for a more effective environmental protection activities from chemical pollutants.

Acknowledgements

This work was supported by grant no. DEC-2013/09/B/NZ9/00226 from the National Science Centre, Poland.

Conflict of interest

Authors declare that there is no conflict of interest that would prejudice the impartiality of this scientific work.

Author details

Malgorzata Duda[1*], Kamil Wartalski[1], Zbigniew Tabarowski[2] and Gabriela Gorczyca[1]

*Address all correspondence to: maja.duda@uj.edu.pl

1 Department of Endocrinology, Institute of Zoology and Biomedical Research, Jagiellonian University in Krakow, Krakow, Poland

2 Department of Experimental Hematology, Institute of Zoology and Biomedical Research, Jagiellonian University in Krakow, Krakow, Poland

References

[1] Walters A, Allan CM, Handelsman DJ. Androgen actions and the ovary. Biology of Reproduction. 2008;**7**:380-389

[2] Weil S, Vendola K, Zhou J, Bondy CA. Androgen and follicle stimulating hormone interactions in primate ovarian follicle development. The Journal of Clinical Endocrinology and Metabolism. 1999;**84**:2951-2956

[3] Yang MY, Fortune JE. Testosterone stimulates the primary to secondary follicles transition in bovine follicles in vitro. Biology of Reproduction. 2006;**75**:924-932

[4] Palacios S. Androgens and female sexual function. The European Menopause Journal. 2007;**57**:61-65

[5] Cardenas H, Jimenez P, Pope WF. Dihydrotestosterone influenced numbers of healthy follicles and follicular amounts of LH receptor mRNA during the follicular phase of the estrous cycle in gilts. Reproduction. 2008;**135**:343-350

[6] Gervásio CG, Bernuci MP, Silva-de-Sá MF, Rosa-E-Silva AC. The role of androgen hormones in early follicular development. ISRN Obstetrics and Gynecology. 2014;**2014**:818010

[7] Zimmermann KC, Bonzon C, Green DR. The machinery of programmed cell death. Pharmacology and Therapeutics. 2001;**92**:57-70

[8] Yu YS, Sui HS, Han ZB, Li W, Luo MJ, Tan JH. Apoptosis in granulosa cell during follicular atresia: Relationship with steroid and insulin-like growth factors. Cell Research. 2004;**14**:341-346

[9] Prizant H, Gleicher N, Sen A. Androgen actions in the ovary: Balance is key. Review Journal of Endocrinology. 2014;**222**:R141-R151

[10] Tetsuka M, Hillier SG. Androgen receptor gene expression in rat granulosa cells: The role of follicle stimulating hormone and steroid hormones. Endocrinology. 1995;**137**:4392-4397

[11] Tetsuka M, Hillier SG. Differential regulation of aromatase and androgen receptor in granulosa cells. The Journal of Steroid Biochemistry and Molecular Biology. 1997;**61**:233-239

[12] Vendola KA, Zhou J, Adesanya OO, Weil SJ, Bondy CA. Androgens stimulate early stages of follicular growth in the primate ovary. The Journal of Clinical Investigation. 1998;**101**:2622-2629

[13] Turner K J, Macpherson S, Millar SM, McNeilly AS, Williams K, et al. Development and validation of a new monoclonal antibody to mammalian aromatase. Journal of Endocrinology. 2002;**172**:21-30

[14] Gunnarsson L. Evolutionary conservation of human drug targets in organisms used for environmental risk assessments. Environmental Science and Technology. 2008;**42**:5807-5813

[15] Hecker M, Holler H. Endocrine disruptor screening: Regulatory perspectives and needs. Environmental Science Europe. 2011;**23**:1-14

[16] Schug TT, Janesick A, Blumberg B, Heindel JJ. Endocrine disrupting chemicals and disease susceptibility. Journal of Steroid Biochemistry and Molecular Biology. 2011;**127**:204-215

[17] Woodruff TK, Walker CL. Fetal and early postnatal environmental exposures and reproductive health effects in the female. Fertility and Sterility. 2008;**89**:e47-e51

[18] Uzumcu M, Zama AM, Oruc E. Epigenetic mechanisms in the actions of endocrine-disrupting chemicals: Gonadal effects and role in female reproduction. Reproduction in Domestic Animals. 2012;**47**:338-347

[19] Maravelias C, Dona A, Stefanidou A, Spiliopoulou C. Adverse effects of anabolic steroids in athletes: A constant threat. Toxicology Letters. 2005;**158**:167-175

[20] Liljeqvist S, Helldén A, Bergman U, Söderberg M. Pulmonary embolism associated with the use of anabolic steroids. European Journal of Internal Medicine. 2008;**19**:214-215

[21] Björnström L, Sjöberg M. Mechanisms of estrogen receptor signaling: Convergence of genomic and nongenomic actions on target genes. Molecular Endocrinology. 2005;**19**:833-842

[22] Lubahn DB, Brown TR, Simental JA, Higgs HN, Migeon CJ, et al. Sequence of the intron/exon junctions of the coding region of the human androgen receptor gene and identification of a point mutation in a family with complete androgen insensitivity. Proceedings of the National Academy of Sciences USA. 1989;**86**:9534-9538

[23] Brockschmidt FF, Nothen MM, Hillmer AM. The two most common alleles of the coding GGN repeat in the androgen receptor gene cause differences in protein function. Journal of Molecular Endocrinology. 2007;**39**:1-8

[24] Buchanan G, Yang M, Cheong A, Harris JM, Irvine RA, et al. Structural and functional consequences of glutamine tract variation in the androgen receptor. Human Molecular Genetics. 2004;**13**:1677-1692

[25] Beato M, Klug J. Steroid hormone receptors: An update. Human Reproduction Update. 2000;**6**:225-236

[26] Kumar R, Thompson EB. Transactivation functions of the N-terminal domains of nuclear hormone receptors: Protein folding and coactivator interactions. Molecular Endocrinology. 2003;**17**:1-10

[27] Matias PM, Donner P, Coelho R, Thomaz M, Peixoto C. Structural evidence for ligand specificity in the binding domain of the human androgen receptor. Implications for pathogenic gene mutations. Journal of Biological Chemistry. 2000;**275**:26164-26171

[28] He B, Gampe RT, Kole AJ, Hnat AT, Stanley TB, et al. Structural basis for androgen receptor interdomain and co-activator interactions suggests a transition in nuclear receptor activation function dominance. Molecular Cell. 2004;**16**:425-438

[29] Shaffer PL, Jivan A, Dollins DE, Claessens F, Gewirth DT. Structural basis of androgen receptor binding to selective androgen response elements. Proceedings of the National Academy of Sciences USA. 2004;**101**:4758-4763

[30] Haelens A, Tanner T, Denayer S, Callewaert L, Claessens F. The hinge region regulates DNA binding, nuclear translocation, and transactivation of the androgen receptor. Cancer Research. 2007;**67**:4514-4523

[31] Ferro P, Catalano MG, Dell'Eva R, Fortunati N, Pfeffer U. The androgen receptor CAG repeat: A modifier of carcinogenesis? Molecular and Cellular Endocrinology. 2002;**193**:109-120

[32] Ding D, Xu L, Menon M, Reddy GP, Barrack ER. Effect of a short CAG (glutamine) repeat on human androgen receptor function. Prostate. 2004;**58**:23-32

[33] Ding D, Xu L, Menon M, Reddy GP, Barrack ER. Effect of GGC (glycine) repeat length polymorphism in the human androgen receptor on androgen action. Prostate. 2005;**62**:133-139

[34] Jenster G, van der Korput HA, Trapman J, Brinkmann AO. Identification of two transcription activation units in the N-terminal domain of the human androgen receptor. The Journal of Biological Chemistry. 1995;**270**:341-7346

[35] Rochette-Egly C. Nuclear receptors: Integration of multiple signalling pathways through phosphorylation. Cell Signalling. 2003;**15**:355-366

[36] Khorasanizadeh S, Rastinejad F. Nuclear-receptor interactions on DNA-response elements. Trends in Biochemical Sciences. 2001;**26**:384-390

[37] Bunone G, Briand PA, Miksicek RJ, Picard D. Activation of the unliganded estrogen receptor by EGF involves the MAP kinase pathway and direct phosphorylation. European Molecular Biology Organization Journal. 1996;**15**:2174-2183

[38] Picard D, Bunone G, Liu JW, Donzé O. Steroid-independent activation of steroid receptors in mammalian and yeast cells and in breast cancer. Biochemical Society Transactions. 1997;**25**:597-602

[39] Simons K, Toomre D. Lipid rafts and signal transduction. Nature Reviews Molecular Cell Biology. 2000;**1**:31-39

[40] Braun A, Thomas P. Biochemical characterization of a membrane androgen receptor in the ovary of the Atlantic croaker. Biology of Reproduction. 2004;**71**:146-155

[41] Thomas P, Dressing G, Pang Y, Berg H, Tubbs C, et al. Progestin, estrogen and androgen G-protein coupled receptors in fish gonads. Steroids. 2006;**71**:310-316

[42] Pi M, Parrill AL, Quarles LD. GPRC6A mediates the non-genomic effects of steroids. Journal of Biological Chemistry. 2010;**285**:39953-39964

[43] Pascal LE, Wang Z. Unzipping androgen action through ZIP9: A novel membrane androgen receptor. Endocrinology. 2014;**155**:4120-4123

[44] Dehm SM, Tindall DJ. Molecular regulation of androgen action in prostate cancer. Journal of Cellular Biochemistry. 2006;**99**:333-344

[45] Liao RS, Ma S, Miao L, Li R, Yin Y, Raj GV. Androgen receptor-mediated non-genomic regulation of prostate cancer cell proliferation. Translational Andrology and Urology. 2013;**2**:187-196

[46] Falkenstein E, Tillmann HC, Christ M, Feuring M, Wehling MC. Multiple actions of steroid hormones – A focus on rapid, nongenomic effects. Pharmacological Review. 2000;**52**:513-556

[47] Cato AC, Nestl A, Mink S. Rapid actions of steroid receptors in cellular signaling pathways. Science's Signal Transduction Knowledge Environment. 2002;**2002**:re9

[48] Dehm SM, Tindall DJ. Alternatively spliced androgen receptor variants. Endocrine-Related Cancer. 2011;**18**:R183-R196

[49] Modrek B, Lee C. A genomic view of alternative splicing. Nature Genetics. 2002;**30**:13-19

[50] Keren H, Lev-Maor G, Ast G. Alternative splicing and evolution: Diversification, exon definition and function. Nature Reviews Genetics. 2010;**11**:345-355

[51] Liu LL, Xie N, Sun S, Plymate S, Mostaghel E, et al. Mechanisms of the androgen receptor splicing in prostate cancer cells. Oncogene. 2014;**33**:3140-3150

[52] Chen J, Weiss WA. Alternative splicing in cancer: Implications for biology and therapy. Oncogene. 2015;**34**:1-14

[53] Piekiełko-Witkowska A, Nauman A. Alternative splicing and its role in pathologies of the endocrine system. Endokrynologia Polska. 2011;**62**:160-170

[54] Norman RJ, Dewailly D, Legro RS, Hickey TE. Polycystic ovary syndrome. Lancet. 2007;**370**:685-697

[55] Wang F, Pan J, Liu Y, Meng Q, Lv P, et al. Alternative splicing of the androgen receptor in polycystic ovary syndrome. Proceedings of the National Academy of Sciences USA. 2015;**112**:4743-4748

[56] Skinner MK. Regulation of primordial follicle assembly and development. Human Reproduction Update. 2005;**11**:461-471

[57] McLaughlin EA, McIver SC. Awakening the oocyte: Controlling primordial follicle development. Reproduction. 2009;**137**:1-11

[58] Eppig JJ, Wigglesworth K, Pendola FL. The mammalian oocyte orchestrates the rate of ovarian follicular development. Proceedings of the National Academy of Sciences USA. 2002;**99**:2890-2894

[59] Smith P, Wilhelm D, Rodgers RJ. Development of mammalian ovary. Journal of Endocrinology. 2014;**221**:R145-R161

[60] Yang JL, Zhang CP, Li L, Huang L, Ji SY, et al. Testosterone induces redistribution of forkhead box-3a and down-regulation of growth and differentiation factor 9 messenger ribonucleic acid expression at early stage of mouse folliculogenesis. Endocrinology 2010;**151**:774-782

[61] Fowler PA, Anderson RA, Saunders PT, Kinnell H, Mason JI, et al. Development of steroid signaling pathways during primordial follicle formation in the human fetal ovary. The Journal of Clinical Endocrinology and Metabolism. 2011;**96**:1754-1762

[62] Narkwichean A, Jayaprakasan K, Maalouf WE, Hernandez-Medrano JH, Pincott-Allen C, Campbell BK. Effects of dehydroepiandrosterone on *in vivo* ovine follicular development. Human Reproduction. 2014;**29**:146-154

[63] Vendola K, Zhou J, Wang J, Famuyiwa OA, Bievre M, Bondy CA. Androgens promote oocyte insulin-like growth factor I expression and initiation of follicle development in the primate ovary. Biology of Reproduction. 1999;**61**:353-357

[64] Magamage MPS, Zengyo M, Moniruzzaman M, Miyano T. Testosterone induces activation of porcine primordial follicles *in vitro*. Reproductive Medicine and Biology. 2011;**10**:21-30

[65] Rice S, Ojha K, Whitehead S, Mason H. Stage-specific expression of androgen receptor, follicle stimulating hormone receptor, and anti-Mullerian hormone type II receptor in single, isolated human preantral follicles: Relevance to polycystic ovaries. The Journal of Clinical Endocrinology and Metabolism. 2007;**92**:1034-1040

[66] Murray AA, Gosden RG, Allison V, Spears N. Effect of androgens on the development of mouse follicles growing *in vitro*. Journal of Reproduction and Fertility. 1998;**113**:27-33

[67] Wang H, Andoh K, Hagiwara H, Xiaowei L, Kikuchi N, et al. Effect of adrenal and ovarian androgens on type 4 follicles unresponsive to FSH in immature mice. Endocrinology. 2001;**142**:4930-4936

[68] Duda M, Wolna A, Knapczyk-Stwora K, Grzesiak M, Knet M, Tabarowski Z, Slomczynska M. The influence of the antiandrogen-2-hydroxyflutamide on the androgen receptor expression in the porcine ovarian follicles – An *in vitro* study. Reproduction in Domestic Animals. 2013;**48**:454-462

[69] Wartalski K, Hereta M, Gorczyca G, Goch P, Tabarowski Z, Duda M. Androgens Influence on *in vitro* Development of Porcine Preantral Follicles. VIII Ovarian Club, 4-7 November, Paris. Available from: http://oc2016.cme-congresses.com/posters.aspx

[70] Gilchrist RB, Ritter LJ, Armstrong DT. Oocyte-somatic cell interactions during follicle development in mammals. Animal Reproduction Science. 2004;**82**:431-446

[71] Salustri A, Fulop C, Camaion A, Hascall VC. Oocyte–granulosa cell interaction. In: Leung PCK and Adashi EY, editors. The ovary. Elsevier Academic Press, San Diego; 2004. p. 131-43

[72] Yeh S, Tsai MY, Xu Q, Mu XM, Lardy H, et al. Generation and characterization of androgen receptor knockout (ARKO) mice: An *in vitro* model for the study of androgen functions in selective tissues. Proceedings of the National Academy of Sciences USA. 2002;**99**:13498-13503

[73] Chang C, Lee SO, Wang RS, Yeh S, Chang TM. Androgen receptor (AR) physiological roles in male and female reproductive systems: Lessons learned from AR-knockout mice lacking AR in selective cells. Biology of Reproduction. 2013;**89**:21

[74] Hu C, Wang PH, Yeh S, Wang S, Xie C, Xu Q, et al. Subfertility and defective folliculogenesis in female mice lacking androgen receptor. Proceedings of the National Academy of Sciences USA. 2004;**101**:11209-11214

[75] Ecay TW, Powers RD. Differential effects of testosterone and dibutyryl cyclic AMP on the meiotic maturation of mouse oocytes *in vitro*. Journal of Experimental Zoology. 1990;**253**:88-98

[76] Anderiesz C, Trounson AO. The effect of testosterone on the maturation and developmental capacity of murine oocytes *in vitro*. Human Reproduction. 1995;**10**:2377-2381

[77] Starowicz A, Galas J, Duda M, Tabarowski Z, Szoltys M. Effects of testosterone and prolactin on steroidogenesis in post-ovulatory cumuli oophori and on *in vitro* oocyte fertilisation in the rat. Reproduction, Fertility and Development. 2017;**29**:406-418

[78] Suzuki O, Koura O, Noguch Y, Uchio-Yamada K, Matsuda J. Reduced superovulation efficiency by high-dose treatment of dehydroepiandrosterone in mice. Reproduction, Fertility and Development. 2012;**25**:307-307

[79] Cardenas H, Pope WF. Androgen receptor and follicle-stimulating hormone receptor in the pig ovary during the follicular phase of the estrous cycle. Molecular Reproduction and Development. 2002;**62**:92-98

[80] Sen A, Hammes SR. Granulosa cell-specific androgen receptors are critical regulators of ovarian development and function. Molecular Endocrinology. 2010;**24**:1393-1403

[81] Kumari GL, Datta JK, Roy S. Evidence for a role of androgens in the growth and maturation of ovarian follicles in rats. Hormone Research. 1978;**9**:112-120

[82] Hejmej A, Kotula-Balak M, Bilinska B. Antiandrogenic and estrogenic compounds: effect on development and function of male reproductive system. In: Abduljabbar H, editor. Steroids - Clinical Aspect. InTech, Croatia; 2011. p. 51-82

[83] Duda M, Durlej M, Knet M, Knapczyk-Stwora K, Tabarowski Z, Slomczynska M. Does 2-hydroxyflutamide inhibit apoptosis in porcine granulosa cells? – An *in vitro* study. Journal of Reproduction and Development. 2012;**58**:438-444

[84] Kelce WR, Wilson EM. Environmental antiandrogens: Developmental effects, molecular mechanisms, and clinical implications. Journal of Molecular Medicine. 1997;**75**:198-207

[85] Kiparissis Y, Metcafle TL, Balch GC, Metcalfe CD. Effects of the antiandrogens, vinclozolin and cyproterone acetate on gonadal development in the Japanese medaka (Oryzias latipes). Aquatic Toxicology. 2003;**63**:391-403

[86] Kavlock R, Cummings A. Mode of action: Inhibition of androgen receptor function-vinclozolin-induced malformations in reproductive development. Critical Reviews in Toxicology. 2005;**35**:721-726

[87] Kelce WR, Monosson E, Gamcsik MP, Laws SC, Gray LE. Environmental hormone disruptors: Evidence that vinclozolin developmental toxicity is mediated by antiandrogenic metabolites. Toxicology and Applied Pharmacology. 1994;**126**:276-285

[88] van Ravenzwaay B, Kolle SN, Ramirez T, Kamp HG. Vinclozolin: A case study on the identification of endocrine active substance in the past and a future perspective. Toxicology Letters. 2013;**223**:271-279

[89] Guerrero-Bosagna C, Covert TR, Haque MM, Settles M, Nilsson EE, Anway MD, Skinner MK. Epigenetic transgenerational inheritance of vinclozolin induced mouse adult onset disease and associated sperm epigenome biomarkers. Reproductive Toxicology. 2012;**34**:694-707

[90] Buckley J, Willingham E, Agras K, Baskin LS. Embryonic exposure to the fungicide vinclozolin causes virilization of females and alteration of progesterone receptor expression *in vivo*: An experimental study in mice. Environmental Health. 2006;**5**:4

[91] Nilsson EE, Anway MD, Stanfield J, Skinner MK. Transgenerational epigenetic effects of the endocrine disruptor vinclozolin on pregnancies and female adult onset disease. Reproduction. 2008;**135**:713-721

[92] Knet M, Tabarowski Z, Slomczynska M, Duda M. The effects of the environmental antiandrogen vinclozolin on the induction of granulosa cell apoptosis during follicular atresia in pigs. Theriogenology. 2014;**81**:1239-1247

[93] Knet M, Wartalski K, Hoja-Lukowicz D, Tabarowski Z, Slomczynska M, Duda M. Analysis of porcine granulosa cell death signaling pathways induced by vinclozolin. Theriogenology. 2015;**84**:927-939

[94] Bauer ERS, Daxenberger A, Petri T, Sauerwein H, Meyer HHD. Characterization of the affinity of different anabolic and synthetic hormones to the human androgen receptor, human sex hormone binding globulin and to the bovine progestin receptor. Acta Pathologica, Microbiologica et Immunologica Scandinavica. 2001;**108**:838-846

[95] McIntyre BS, Barlow NJ, Wallace DG, Maness SC, Gaido KW, Foster PM. Effects of in utero exposure to linuron on androgen-dependent reproductive development in the male Crl:CD(SD)BR rat. Toxicology and Applied Pharmacology. 2000;**167**:87-99

[96] Hotchkiss AK, Parks-Saldutti LG, Ostby JS, Lambright C, Furr J, et al. A mixture of the "antiandrogens" linuron and butyl benzyl phthalate alters sexual differentiation of the male rat in a cumulative fashion. Biology of Reproduction. 2004;**71**:1852-1861

[97] Turner KJ, McIntyre BS, Phillips SL, Barlow NJ, Bowman CJ, Foster PM. Altered gene expression during rat Wolffian duct development in response to *in utero* exposure to the antiandrogen linuron. Toxicological Science. 2003;**74**:114-128

[98] Wilson VS, Lambright CR, Furr JR, Howdeshell KL, Earl Gray L Jr. The herbicide linuron reduces testosterone production from the fetal rat testis during both *in utero* and *in vitro* exposures. Toxicology Letters. 2009;**186**:73-77

[99] Pregel P, Bollo E, Cannizzo FT, Rampazzo A, Appino S, Biolatti B. Effect of anabolics on bovine granulosa-luteal cell primary cultures. Folia Histochemica et Cytobiologica. 2007;**45**:265-271

[100] Nielsen SW, Kennedy PC. In: Moulton J, editor. Tumors in domestic animals. 3rd ed. Los Angeles CA: University of California Press; 1990. pp. 502-508

[101] Matzuk MM, Burns KH, Viveiros MM, Eppig JJ. Intercellular communication in the mammalian ovary: Oocytes carry the conversation. Science. 2002;**296**:2178-2180

[102] Fortune JE, Ribera GM, Yang MY. Follicular development: The role of follicular microenvironment in selection of dominant follicle. Animal Reproduction Science. 2004;**82**: 109-126

[103] Gibson DA, Simitsidellis I, Collins F, Saunders P. Evidence of androgen action in endometrial and ovarian cancers. Endocrine-Related Cancer. 2014;**21**:203-218

[104] Migliaccio A, Castoria G, Di Domenico M, et al. Sex steroids hormones and growth factors. The Journal of Steroid Biochemistry and Molecular Biology .2002;**83**:31-35

[105] Hsueh AJ, Billig H, Tsafriri A. Ovarian follicle atresia: A hormonally controlled apoptotic process. Endocrine Reviews. 1994;**15**:707-724

[106] Segars JH, Driggers PH. Estrogen action and cytoplasmic signaling cascades. Trends in Endocrinology and Metabolism. 2002;**13**:349-354

[107] De Brabander HF, Poelmans S, Schilt R, et al. Presence and metabolism of the anabolic steroid boldenone in various animal species. A review. Food Additives and Contaminants. 2004;**21**:515-525

[108] Vaiserman A. Early-life exposure to endocrine disrupting chemicals and later-life health outcomes: An epigenetic bridge? Aging Disorders. 2014;**5**:419-429

[109] Patel S, Zhou C, Rattan S, Flaws JA. Effects of endocrine-disrupting chemicals on the ovary. Biology of Reproduction. 2015;**93**:1-9

Chapter 2

Estrus Cycle Monitoring in Wild Mammals: Challenges and Perspectives

Alexandre R. Silva, Nei Moreira,
Alexsandra F. Pereira, Gislayne C.X. Peixoto,
Keilla M. Maia, Lívia B. Campos and Alana A. Borges

Additional information is available at the end of the chapter

http://dx.doi.org/10.5772/intechopen.69444

Abstract

The knowledge of reproductive physiology is of paramount importance to guide reproductive management and to make possible future application of assisted reproduction techniques (ARTs) aiming ex situ conservation of wild mammals. Nevertheless, information on the basic reproductive aspects of wild mammals remain scarce, and appropriate management practices have not yet been developed for all the species. This chapter discusses the methods most currently used for reproductive monitoring in wild females. Additionally, the difficulties regarding their use in different species and the possibilities of these procedures in captivity or in free-living mammals are addressed.

Keywords: wild animals, female reproductive physiology, hormonal profile, noninvasive monitoring, captive management

1. Introduction

Considering that reproduction is an essential process for species survival, the use of assisted reproduction techniques (ARTs) in wild mammals' conservation allows the storage and exchange of genetic material between populations. Nevertheless, conservation initiatives depend on a profound knowledge of the species' reproductive physiology, since it is not always possible, for some endangered species, to extrapolate from domestic species or even from other wild species counterparts [1].

Thus, ARTs will only be successfully applied for conservation after mastering the aspects related to anatomy and physiology, namely, the characteristics of the reproductive cycle, seasonality, behavior, and other general mechanisms that regulate reproduction [2]. An important factor that hinders reproductive monitoring is the lack of knowledge about the reproductive biology of various wild mammals, which makes the knowledge on their reproductive behavior scarce [3]. Even though the observation of external estrus signs can be used for heat detection, it must be associated with other techniques, for example, vaginal cytology, hormone measurement, ultrasonography, or thermography, in order to determine the most appropriate time for mating or artificial insemination.

Thus, this chapter presents the methods most currently used for reproductive assessment in wild females. In addition, the difficulties regarding its use in different species and the possibilities for using these procedures in captivity or in free-living animals are addressed.

2. Reproductive behavior analysis

Behavioral expression is a major aspect of animal communication and easily reflects the reproductive status to other members of the species. Mammals display considerable variation in the display of behaviors during different physiological states. The study of wild animal behavior is essential for implementing captive breeding programs. The lack of knowledge of the species behavior in its natural environment limits our ability to meet their needs in captivity. In this sense, information about changes in their reproductive behavior can be used to aid monitor the cyclicity of wild females [4, 5].

The behavioral patterns can vary accordingly to the different phases of the estrus cycle. Among the female-specific behaviors, restlessness, characteristic vocalization, standing heat, vaginal mucus discharge, reduced milk secretion, and reduced food intake can be more frequent or intense during estrus [6]. In some wild ungulates, females generate signs of sexual receptivity as visually salient sexual swellings, olfactory cues, or copulation calls [7]. In the captive goral (*Naemorhedus griseus*), the most prevalent behavior is tail-up, which generally persists for 2–3 days associated with 35% of estrogen surges, followed by ovulation (based on elevation of progestogens). Captive goral females also performed head butts and whistles [8].

A study linked the behavioral and physiological reproductive patterns during the periovulatory period and beginning of pregnancy in collared peccaries (*Pecari tajacu*). In that study, Silva et al. [9] referred that behavioral monitoring is a useful procedure for recognition of this period, as long as associated to the other morphophysiological parameters and it should be useful for good practices of collared peccaries handling in captivity and for the improvement of ARTs.

Nonetheless, females in other species may have a silent estrus, in which the ovarian activity is not identified by external signs. External estrus signs are quite inconspicuous in elephants (*Elephas maximus*), and it is difficult to assess their estrus cyclicity using physical cues [10]. Even though elephants have a long estrus cycle of 14–16 weeks, the receptive period is relatively short, lasting for 2–10 days. In general, females display their receptive period through discreet chemical, auditory, and behavioral expressions to attract males [11]. Moreover, in elephants, estrus behavior includes getting away from the herd in an arc-shaped trail, presenting its head tilted to the side to attract males or inform its state ("estrus walk"). They vocalize deep roaring sounds, flick their tail against the vulva, lift, and hold it in the air. When chased, female may first run away but eventually will return toward the bull and accept his mounting [12].

In addition, in many species in captivity, the estrus signs are not frequent or easily observed, mainly due to changes of social and natural habits or small enclosures, in addition to the stress caused by visitors, handling, and management [13]. The estrus cycle length in white rhinoceros (*Ceratotherium simum*) lasts from 4 to 10 weeks, but the reason for this variation remains unknown. Under captivity, this species undergoes long anovulatory periods without luteal activity, which are considered a major reason for their low reproductive rate [14].

Regarding wild felids, major estrus behavioral activities described in the domestic cat, as vocalization, rolling, and urine spray or marking, are also observed in Asiatic lion (*Panthera leo persica*). According to Umapathy et al. [15], vocalization was generally followed by rolling. Females immediately after a bout of vocalization rolled 3–4 times on their dorsal side, and the duration ranged from 10 to 30 s. The frequency of behavioral display is increased on the third day and decreased on the 6th day of estrus. Rubbing of the body against objects and lordosis were also observed during estrus in this species, alike in other small felid species (ocelots, tigrinas, and margays). Moreover, females may show restlessness, an increased frequency of urination (in small quantities), vocalization, and sexual receptivity reactions in the presence of the male, as well as courting acceptance [15].

Scoring of genital appearance, particularly if using digital cameras, is a noninvasive method that provides valuable information and does not require additional training time, laboratory work, or extra expense. Studies were carried out in sun bears (*Helarctos malayanus*) using video-recorded females to evaluate estrus behavior related to other parameters. The vulvar swelling and color were correlated; nevertheless, vulvar swelling appeared to be a more discriminating indicator of estrus. During the 4 days of interval before the estrogen peak, female bears in this study had more agonistic behavior, displayed noticeable declines in appetite, showed more vulvar opening, and increased the number of superficial and keratinized cells in vaginal cytology. At the estrogen peak (day 0 of estrus), a high number of superficial cells were observed, coincident with open vulva, a decrease in agonistic behavior, an increase in affiliate behaviors, and low appetite. In addition, sexual behavior occurred until 4 days after the estrogen peak, along with vaginal keratinized cells and presumably overlapped with ovulation [16]. The study not only confirmed the utility of behavioral measures but also showed that a simple keeper check sheet can be a valuable auxiliary tool for reproductive assessment, offering an alternative to data laboriously derived from video-scored recordings.

Matschie's tree kangaroo (*Dendrolagus matschiei*) is the predominant species of tree kangaroo held in North American zoos [17]. Importation of individuals from the wild is restricted, and, therefore, the captive population must be sustainable through oriented reproduction. Males and females are generally held separately in captivity and paired for mating during estrus, which is identified through observation of proceptive behaviors, for example, licking of the forearms and affiliation with males. Additional information on tree kangaroo's reproductive biology is needed to advance captive propagation of this endangered species. In this sense, noninvasive techniques that eliminate blood collection associated stress are very welcome to study its reproduction [17].

Taking into account the importance of the knowledge of the reproductive behavior of wild animals as a method of estrus cycle monitoring, the main difficulties are especially the lack of knowledge on the physiology and behavior of various wild species in captivity. The perspectives of using this method associated with other noninvasive techniques are good, since it is increasingly necessary to minimize the stress associated with the management of captive animals and to affect as little as possible its reproductive function.

3. External features and vaginal cytology

The focus of an effective estrus detection is to determine the optimal time for mating and the ideal time for artificial insemination. Among the many methods available to identify the estrus cycle, the observation of external estrus signs and vaginal cytology is highlighted. In vaginal cytology (**Figure 1**), the epithelial cell morphology reflects the effect of the interaction of various hormones, particularly estrogen and progesterone, on the reproductive tract. Since the vaginal epithelium reflects the changes in hormone milieu, it follows that any abnormality in the sexual cycle due to either a direct hormonal involvement or disease condition would be reflected in changes in the cell types of vaginal epithelium. Additionally, this technique is simple, practical, economically viable, and in some wild mammal species can be used for characterizing the estrus cycle [18].

In elephants, the use of vaginal cytology has been described since the 1970s by Jainudeen et al. [19] and Watson and D'Souza [20], who described the smear from the vaginal vestibule or vagina in this species. In fact, gathering a vaginal vestibule smear from an elephant is relatively easy if the zoo conducts "free contact" animal training on a regular basis, which facilitates the monitoring of the estrus cycle [21]. A subsequent study conducted in elephants used a spectrum analysis, the Yule-Walker method, to verify the frequency of exfoliative cells. It was found that the markedly appearance of nucleated and enucleated superficial cells characterized the periods from proestrus to estrus, while an increase of intermediate and parabasal cells characterized the period from metestrus to diestrus [21]. In addition, other estrus signs include mucus droppings and the reddening and exposition of the clitoris and the emission of infrasonic sounds and olfactory chemicals, which can be transmitted over greater distances as verified both for Asian [22] and African individuals [23].

In wild carnivores, as the maned wolf (*Chrysocyon brachyurus*), the vaginal cytology is an effective procedure to determine the estrus cycle phases, but, unlike the domestic dogs, blood cells were scarce in all phases of the estrus cycle, including proestrus [24]. Furthermore, these findings may be associated with visible signs of estrus, which are characterized as swelling of the vulva and rosy or bloody vaginal secretions at the beginning of estrus. Already at the end of estrus, the vaginal secretion changes to a thick and yellowish appearance [25].

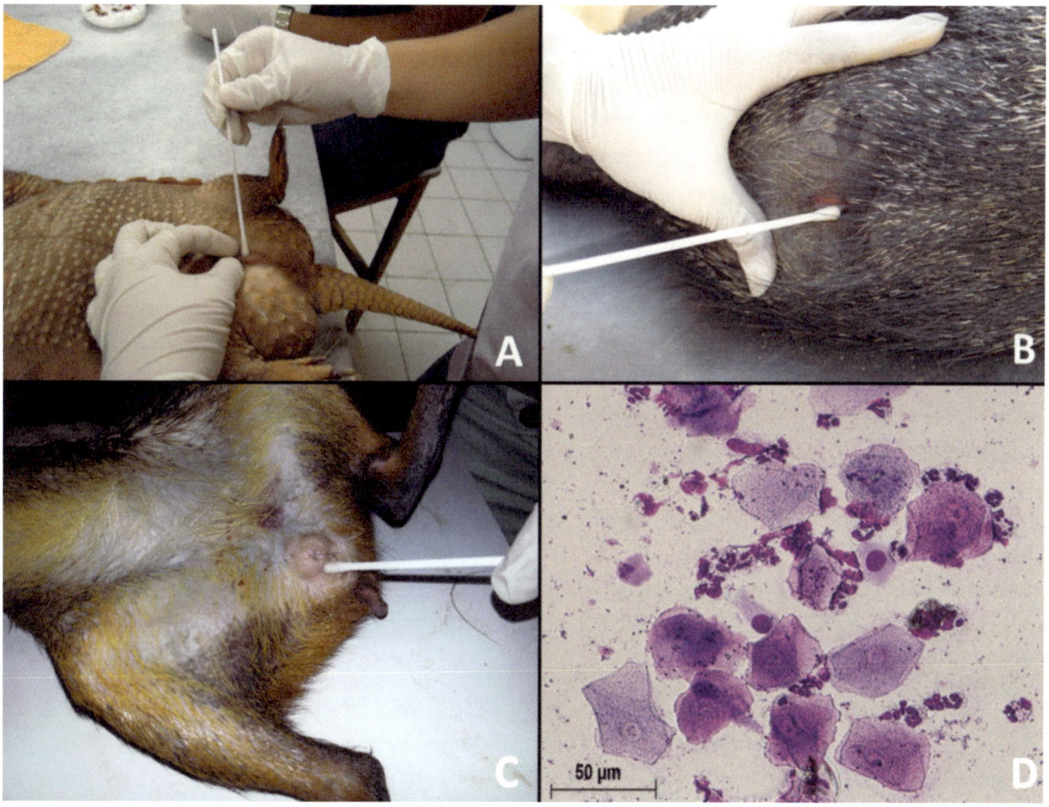

Figure 1. Collection of vaginal smears using swabs from female armadillo, *Euphractus sexcinctus* (A); collared peccary, *Pecari tajacu* (B); and agouti, *Dasyprocta leporina* (C). Cytological specimen presenting predominance of cornified cells indicating estrus in *E. sexcinctus* (D).

The reproduction in captive wild felids, even in relatively naturalistic enclosures, remains poor, especially in small species, which seem to be more susceptible to stress. Puma (*Puma concolor*) females vocalize characteristically during estrus, while ocelots show more estrus signs than other small felid species. In general, females rarely exhibit regular overt signs of sexual receptivity as a higher frequency of rubbing, vocalizing, rolling, urine spraying, and sniffing. These characteristics have been described in Siberian tigers (*Panthera tigris altaica*) [26], clouded leopard (*Neofelis nebulosa*) [27], and *Leopardus* genus [28]. For this reason, the detection of estrus by vaginal cytology is a resource in their reproductive evaluation but requires physical and/or chemical contention. In addition, this method has been described for lions (*Panthera leo*) [29], cheetahs (*Acinonyx jubatus*) [30], pumas [31], and ocelots (*Leopardus pardalis*) [32] in which the estrus was characterized by the presence of a high percentage of keratinized superficial cells.

In sun bears (*H. malayanus*), the vaginal cytology, vulvar changes, and behavior were essential for the characterization of the estrus cycle. Sexual behavior characteristics of estrus include self-masturbation; the interaction among partners, including mutual genital grooming, genital inspect, mount and copulate, affiliative (social play, solicit, follow, groom, and muzzle-muzzle contact), and stereotyped (pacing and other repetitive movements) behaviors, which are displayed along with changes in genital appearance (as vulva color and swell); and the presence of superficial and keratinized cells in vaginal cytology. These characteristics are effective and inexpensive supplements or alternatives to fecal hormone assays and are highly recommended for the continued reproductive management of this and other captive bear populations [33].

Observations of changes in the external genitalia, as the presence of vaginal mucus, hyperemic vaginal mucosa, and separation of the vulvar lips, are also important for estrus identification in collared peccaries [34]. Regarding the use of vaginal cytology for estrus monitoring in this species, Guimarães et al. [35] suggested that it is possible to differentiate estrus cycle stages using this technique. Even though superficial and intermediate cells are present in higher numbers throughout the estrus cycle, the superficial ones significantly increase during the estrus. Nevertheless, authors highlighted that for the correct identification of estrus phases, it is necessary to consider other aspects, as the presence or absence of leukocytes and the relation between the number of intermediate and superficial cells, besides the signs of external genitalia. Conversely, Maia et al. [34] suggested that no significant differences between proportions of vaginal epithelial cells were identified when comparing follicular and luteal phases in collared peccaries. Therefore, an association is suggested among vaginal cytology, behavior and external genitalia observation, and ultrasound and hormonal analysis for correct estrus detection in this species.

Despite the relative success of vaginal cytology described above, it is not always possible to distinguish among the phases of estrus cycle. In Xenarthras, as the maned sloths (*Bradypus torquatus*), this technique was used only to identify estrus, being characterized by the predominance of nucleated and enucleated superficial cells [36]. Moreover, in six-banded armadillos (*Euphractus sexcinctus*), the use of vaginal cytology is difficult because it requires the use of an anesthetic protocol due to their small vulvar commissure that hinders the swab introduction. Nevertheless, this technique does not allow a detailed identification of all phases of estrus cycle, being only possible to distinguish between the follicular and the luteal phase [37]. In fact, alterations in external genitalia seem to be very effective for estrus monitoring in Xenarthras. Both in *Tamandua* (*Tamandua tetradactyla*) [38] and in six-banded armadillos [37, 39], the presence of a vulvar bleeding was used as the main parameter to identify the beginning of the estrus cycle. Moreover, in armadillos, the presence of vulvar bleeding occurred approximately 3–7 days after estrogen rise, concomitant to the presence of vulvar edema and mucus [37]. In this species, the occurrence of clitoral hyperemia, varying between red and purple, and a pronounced clitoral erection was also described [39].

Some difficulties in the use of vaginal cytology for a detailed identification of the stages of estrus cycle have also been described for various wild rodents, as coypus (*Myocastor coypus*) [40], chinchillas (*Chinchilla lanigera*) [41], pacas (*Agouti paca*) [42], and agoutis (*Dasyprocta agouti*) [43]. The main reason for such difficulty is the existence of a vaginal occlusion membrane that tends to obstruct the external vaginal ostium, which remains until the estrus or parturition. The observation of vaginal opening, in parallel with the exfoliative cytology [44], allows the correct identification of estrus in *D. agouti* [43], *Dasyprocta prymnolopha* [45], *Cavia porcellus* [46], *Myoprocta pratti* [47], and chinchillas [48]. As an exception, the use of vaginal cytology in the Spix's yellow-toothed cavy (*Galea spixii*) is reported to be very effective to distinguish the phases of the estrus cycle. In these rodents, a predominance of large intermediate cells is observed in proestrus, while superficial cells predominate in estrus, and the intermediate and parabasal cells prevail in diestrus [49].

The use of vaginal cytology has also been reported for common wombat (*Vombatus ursinus*), but the cycle stages are not accurately identified due to the high variability in the proportion of epithelial cells obtained in the smear analysis [50, 51]. In addition, the anatomy of the urogenital sinus, whose length varies between individuals and within an individual at different cycle stages [50], hinders the collection of an adequate cytological specimen [52]. As the vaginal swab collection procedure requires anesthesia in this species, repeated capture of the female wombat for sequential analysis is likely to be highly stressful, leading to potential reproductive failure [51]. As a marsupial, the condition of the pouch, namely, its depth, opening size, wall thickness, degree of cleanliness, and teat length, could also be indicatives for the reproductive status of wombats (i.e., whether cycling or not) [52, 53]. Alternatively, the observation of the external genitalia changes (clitoris and pericloacal region) that can become swollen and tumescent in different stages of the cycle was proposed for assessing the wombats' reproductive status [53]. However, this technique is not reliable due to the difficulty in detecting any noticeable genitalia changes [52]. An interesting study, conducted by Hogan et al. [54], showed that estrus was not detectable in female southern hairy-nosed wombat (*Lasiorhinus latifrons*) even when the continuous observations of physical activity via movement-sensitive transmitters were used. No difference in physical activity was recorded during estrus and anestrus, or there was any correlation between physical activity and the occurrence of reproductive behavior. In fact, even though numerous studies have examined Vombatidae reproductive behavior, estrus has rarely been observed and appears to be exceptionally short, as 15 h in the common wombat [55] or 13 h in the southern hairy-nosed wombat [56]. The reason why estrus is so short in wombats has yet to be determined. Further studies into reliable methods of estrus detection are urgently required, as the lack of specific information might be the most significant impediment to successfully breeding this species in captivity [57].

In general, the association between the vaginal cytology techniques and the observation of external estrus signs are useful for estrus cycle monitoring in various wild females. Thus, the ability to assess in an easy and safe way the reproductive status through noninvasive means is vital to understand the reproductive physiology of animals. Therefore, such methods ought to contribute to assist captive breeding of threatened species, additionally, in order to ensure better reproductive performance in animal production and the development of techniques and tools for assisted reproduction.

4. Endocrine monitoring and its metabolites

Endocrine monitoring enables the knowledge of endocrine activity as a tool to evaluate the ovarian cycle and to be used in a captive management, especially for endangered species, aiming to increase the number of individuals [58]. In wild mammals, the endocrine monitoring of the estrus cycle can either be performed by invasive methods, as using blood samples [59], or noninvasive methods, by sampling from feces [8], urine [60], saliva [61], and hair [62].

The choice of the hormonal monitoring method depends on the type of assessment method selected (invasive and noninvasive) and on the requested information, as well as on the differences among species, hormone metabolism, excretion pathway, and viability during collection and processing [63]. In either method, the main analysis procedures available include the immunoassay, as enzyme immunoassay (EIA) [8], radioimmunoassay (RIA), and chemiluminescence [64], with antibodies directed to the hormone of interest [11] and also high-performance liquid chromatography (HPLC) [65].

In general, endocrine monitoring in wild mammals has been carried out in blood samples for species that do not suffer so much stress during collection, as Elephantidae [58]. Already feces, urine, saliva, and hair were used in Cervidae [66], Rhinocerotidae [67], Felidae [28], and Ursidae [68].

4.1. Blood samples

Among the type of samples, the blood is the one that promotes a faster response to the endocrine cycle, also making possible to extrapolate the evaluation of steroids, for proteins, luteinizing hormone (LH), follicle-stimulating hormone (FSH), inhibin, prolactin, and relaxin [69]. The invasive method by blood sampling has the advantage of providing more immediate and accurate information regarding the peripheral hormone levels [58]. After collection, the blood is centrifuged to obtain serum or plasma that can be stored at −20°C until analysis [11].

This method has been used in armadillos, collared peccaries, elephants, and agoutis. In armadillos, a clear identification of a 23.5 days of estrus cycle was made, consisting of 8.8 days for follicular and 15.6 days for luteal phase [37]. In collared peccaries, the estrus cycle lasts 21 days, with a follicular phase of 6 days and 15 days for the luteal phase [34]. In Asian elephants, the estrus cycle has an overall duration of 12–19 weeks, the luteal phase extending between 4 and 15 weeks, and the follicular phase lengthening for 2–12 weeks [11]. In red-rumped agoutis, the estrus cycle lasts for 31 days, the follicular phase ranging from 6 to 9 days, and the luteal phase from 19 to 23 days [59].

Nevertheless, this method has the inconvenience of causing a high level of stress in several wild mammals, associated with blood sampling, whose collection needs a more laborious procedure, as physical and chemical contention of the animal [37]. Moreover, the generated stress can result in a change in hormonal levels [64]. Additionally, the blood collection requires the training of the operator that will collect the sample, besides the adaptation of the animal to this type of management [58]. Thus, although the blood samples are quite sensitive to hormonal changes and allow the evaluation of a greater number of hormones, in wild mammals it is preferable to use noninvasive methods, so to avoid contact with the animal and reduce stress into a minimum.

In addition to animal stress, difficulties and risks associated with blood collection and sometimes training requirements supported the development of alternative methods for hormonal assessment. In this sense, noninvasive methods have the advantage of an easy collection of the sample, without causing stress to the animal. These methods assume that hormones that circulate in the bloodstream are secreted into the saliva, deposited in the hair, and excreted via feces or urine [63]. Nevertheless, it has the disadvantages that the immunogenic form of hormones in urine and feces is different in some species, because they are metabolized in the liver and kidney, mainly in a biologically inactive form [58].

4.2. Fecal samples

In general, fecal steroid metabolites are the most common noninvasive method to screen the endocrine function in wild mammals, allowing the knowledge of the reproductive biology of several species. The metabolic pathway involves the inactivation or excretion of hormones and metabolites of steroids that have different routes according to species and the type of steroid in the same species [63]. The main estrogen metabolites present in fecal samples are estrone, estradiol-17α, and estradiol-17β [70]. Already progesterone metabolites present in fecal samples are allopregnanolone (5α-P-3OH) [10], 17a-hydroxyprogesterone [15], and pregnanediol-3-glucuronide (PdG) [71]. The fecal samples have a pattern of steroid concentration similar to the one found in plasma, with a delay in relation to blood due to metabolism and excretion (lag time), which can vary from hours to days depending on the species [63].

The collection of fecal samples is simple; nevertheless, the preparation of this sample requires a longer time. This type of sample should be stored at −20°C because of the presence of gastrointestinal bacteria that can degrade the hormones and cause changes in concentrations [27]. Subsequently, fecal samples need to be homogenized prior to the steroid uniformity, the extraction in the presence of methanol or ethanol, and the evaluation of hormones in the supernatant after centrifugation [72]. Steroid and prostaglandin metabolites are lipophilic and are usually conjugated in the liver to soluble portions for excretion into feces [73].

The enzyme immunoassay for monitoring fecal metabolites has been successfully used in wild felid species, as ocelots, tigrinas (*Leopardus tigrinus*), and margays (*Leopardus wiedii*), allowing to determine the mean length of the estrus cycle as 18.4, 16.7, and 17.6 days, respectively [28]. Results derived from hormonal assessment in feces from several other wild mammals are reported in **Table 1**.

4.3. Urine samples

In most cases, fecal analysis can measure estradiol-17β, estrone conjugates (E1C), progesterone, and PdG, whereas urine analysis (**Table 1**) is generally used to measure E1C and PdG [71]. Moreover, peptide hormones can be filtered through the renal glomerulus and excreted in urine [64]. Analysis of urinary hormones or their metabolites in many cetacean species has been successful in detecting estrus, developing the ability to define patterns of endocrine excretion [60].

In general, urine collection requires proper training of the animal, to avoid contamination of the samples [61]. In case of untrained animals, this material is collected on the ground, and it is necessary to isolate the animal, which causes stress besides requiring a time for the isolation and urine recovery [58]. These uses of urine samples also require a previous step, that is, creatinine

Samples	Species	Metabolites	Hormonal assay	Follicular phase	Luteal phase	Ovarian cycle	References
Fecal	*Myrmecophaga tridactyla*	E2/P4	EIA/HPCL	34.5 d	16.9 d	51.4 d	Patzl et al. [77]
Fecal	*Naemorhedus griseus*	E2/P4	EIA	3 d	18 d	21 d	Khonmee et al. [8]
Fecal	*Gorilla beringei beringei*	E2/P4	EIA/LC-MS/HPLC	21 d	8 d	29 d	Habumuremyi et al. [65]
Fecal	*Rhinoceros unicornis*	E2/P4	EIA/HPCL	15.9 d	19.1 d	43.4 d	Schwarzenberger et al. [67]
Fecal	*Ceratotherium simum*	20-oxo-P	EIA/HPCL	12.4 d	55.9 d	68.3 d	Schwarzenberger et al. [78]
Fecal	*Tragulus javanicus*	E2/P4	EIA/HPCL	11.5 d	3 d	14.5 d	Kusuda et al. [72]
Fecal	*Perodicticus potto*	E2/P4	EIA	9.1 d	19.89 d	36.06 d	MacKinnon et al. [79]
Urine/fecal	*Rhinopithecus roxellana*	E2G/PdG/E2/PdG	EIA	14.7 d	10.4 d	25.1 d	Muren et al. [71]
Urine	*Delphinapterus leucas*	E2/P4	EIA/HPCL	25 d	25 d	50 d	Steinman et al. [60]
Urine	*Tursiops truncatus*	EC/LH/UP	EIA/UP/HPLC	8 d	19 d	27 d	Robeck et al. [80]
Urine	*Lagenorhynchus obliquidens*	EC/LH/UP	EIA/UP/HPLC	10 d	21 d	31 d	Robeck et al. [81]
Saliva	*Loxodonta africana*	P4	EIA	4.6 wk	18.6 wk	23.2 wk	Illera et al. [61]
Saliva	*Trichechus inunguis*	E2/P4	EIA	19 d	27.33 d	47.67 d	Amaral et al. [75]

Saliva and fecal samples were stored at −20°C and urine samples at −70°C.

Abbreviations: enzyme immunoassay (EIA), liquid chromatography-mass spectrometry (LC-MS), high-performance liquid chromatography (HPLC), estradiol-17β (E2), progesterone (P4), total immunoreactive 20-oxo-pregnanes (20-oxo-P), estradiol-3-glucuronide (E2G), pregnanediol-3-glucuronide (PdG), estrogen conjugates (EC), luteinizing hormone (LH), urinary progesterone (UP) metabolites, day (d), week (wk).

Table 1. Monitoring the ovarian cycle of some wild mammals using noninvasive methods.

analysis to evaluate if the sample is much diluted for subsequent hormonal evaluation [74]. It also includes centrifugation for separation of particles that can cause contamination.

Urine samples can be stored for 24 h at room temperature; if there is an interest in measuring proteo- or peptide hormones, it is advisable to freeze the sample since these particles are easily degraded. For the gonadotrophins analysis, it is usual to add glycerol in the sample, to avoid dissociation in subunits. On the other hand, sex steroid hormones are secreted as conjugates soluble in water [63]; estrone (E1) and PdG represent the urinary metabolites of estradiol and progesterone, respectively, in most primate species [71].

4.4. Saliva samples

The sex steroid hormones found in saliva retain the same form as in blood because circulating steroid hormones pass through the epithelium of exocrine glands by passive diffusion [75]. Thus, the saliva becomes the suitable sample for endocrine monitoring, since it has unaltered steroid and whole peptide hormones [64]. In relation to the hormonal proportions of the blood in the saliva, it is possible to detect a smaller amount of steroid and peptide/proteo-hormones [63]. The saliva reflects the hormonal changes in the blood, allowing for its immediate analysis [61]. The hormonal levels in saliva have a difficult interpretation since this is easily changed in a short period [75]. Moreover, as the hormones detected in saliva are quite similar to the blood, these suffer less the specific species effect, allowing the use of commercial kits [63].

Salivary samples are obtained with the aid of swab and stored at −20°C. In addition, the samples can be previously lyophilized or simply centrifuged and suspended in buffer for subsequent EIA [61]. Nevertheless, the method is still seldom used because of the difficulty in collection that requires a closer contact to the animal to obtain the sample [66], being performed in few species (**Table 1**).

4.5. Hair samples

The hair can also be used as a source for measuring hormone levels, since through the bloodstream, hormones are deposited in the hair follicle [62]. The hair is considered as a form of long-term monitoring because it will detect endocrine activity for months or weeks and will not represent hormone levels for hours or days; nevertheless, the hormones are structurally similar to the forms found in blood [76].

In Canada lynx (*Lynx canadensis*), the hormone measurements from hair samples are foreseen as a promising method for reproductive surveillance; nevertheless, it still requires more studies and validation to be reliable and widely applied [62]. In general, the hair is pre-washed with methanol, collected with commercial clippers, and stored at room temperature in aluminum foil until analysis. In primates, the use of hair to measure the hormonal exposure of fetuses was possible through mass spectrometry (MS) and high-performance liquid chromatography (HPLC), demonstrating that this method has the ability to predict hormone levels [76]. Although the method of endocrine monitoring via hair is very interesting for the knowledge of the estrus cycle, further studies are necessary, because this method is more directed to the measurement of cortisol levels [64].

In summary, the availability of different methods of endocrine monitoring in wild animals makes it possible to choose the most appropriate method for the species of interest, considering the hormonal metabolism and the metabolite evaluated. Although some species allow blood collection, for most wild mammals, noninvasive methods are preferable to minimize stress during collection. This knowledge of the endocrine mechanism concurs to the conservation of wild mammals, fostering the study of species of unknown physiology and the assessment of endocrine profiles in reproductive biotechnology. Therefore, the endocrine monitoring is an important tool to study hormonal ovarian activity of wild mammals.

5. Ultrasonography

Ultrasonography is a classical and reliable method for monitoring ovarian dynamic in mammals (**Figure 2**). In wild females, ultrasound is an integral part of ART procedures allowing the monitoring of sexual cycles. Moreover, ultrasound aids to confirm the efficiency of estrus synchronization and superovulation protocols and to identify the presence of follicles and corpora lutea and the follow up of follicular dynamics [82]. In addition, ultrasound can assist in the study of corpus luteum regression mechanisms, thus allowing to confirm the response to hormonal treatments for estrus control. Nevertheless, the effective application of ultrasound varies among different species, being dependent of several characteristics, as ovary size [83].

Follicles within the ovaries appear as anechoic spherical structures, while the corpus luteum appears with distinctive margins and non-smooth surfaces that are hypoechoic or anechoic in the center, presenting homogeneous fluid dark spaces. This description, observed in the majority of mammalian species, can be extrapolated for wild animals [84].

Among nonhuman primates, the initial studies in the common marmoset (*Callithrix jacchus*) showed that ultrasound provides a reliable and noninvasive method for ovarian cycle evaluation. The cycles were monitored by plasma progesterone, and ultrasound reliability was validated by comparing the findings with direct observation of the ovaries (number and position of structures) through laparotomy. In those animals, 92% of the follicles and 78% of corpus luteum were correctly determined by ultrasound [85]. In capuchin monkeys (*Sapajus paella*), the dominant follicle was recognized at 6 days prior to ovulation with the use of 2D ultrasound, the diameter and mean volume of preovulatory follicle being estimated as 9.6 mm and 0.54 mL, respectively [86]. By ultrasound, the occurrence of ovulation was observed when the mean diameter of the ovulatory follicle was 9 mm, the follicle size being an important parameter to estimate the ovulation day in this species [87].

For ungulates as cervids, the transrectal ultrasonography has been described for evaluating the ovarian response in wapitis (*Cervus elaphus*) subjected to estrus synchronization protocol (CIDR-B, 1.9 g of progesterone and 200 IU of eCG) used for fixed-time artificial insemination (FTAI). In this occasion, corpus luteum and ovulatory follicles (≥8 mm) were easily detected [88]. In Jilin sika deer (*Cervus nippon hortulorum*), the transrectal ultrasonography enabled the consistent visualization of both ovaries and allowed the detailed characterization of follicular dynamics during the estrus cycle. In this species, it has been shown that the follicular wave started with a follicle with ≥4 mm diameter, and it ended in the day when the number of

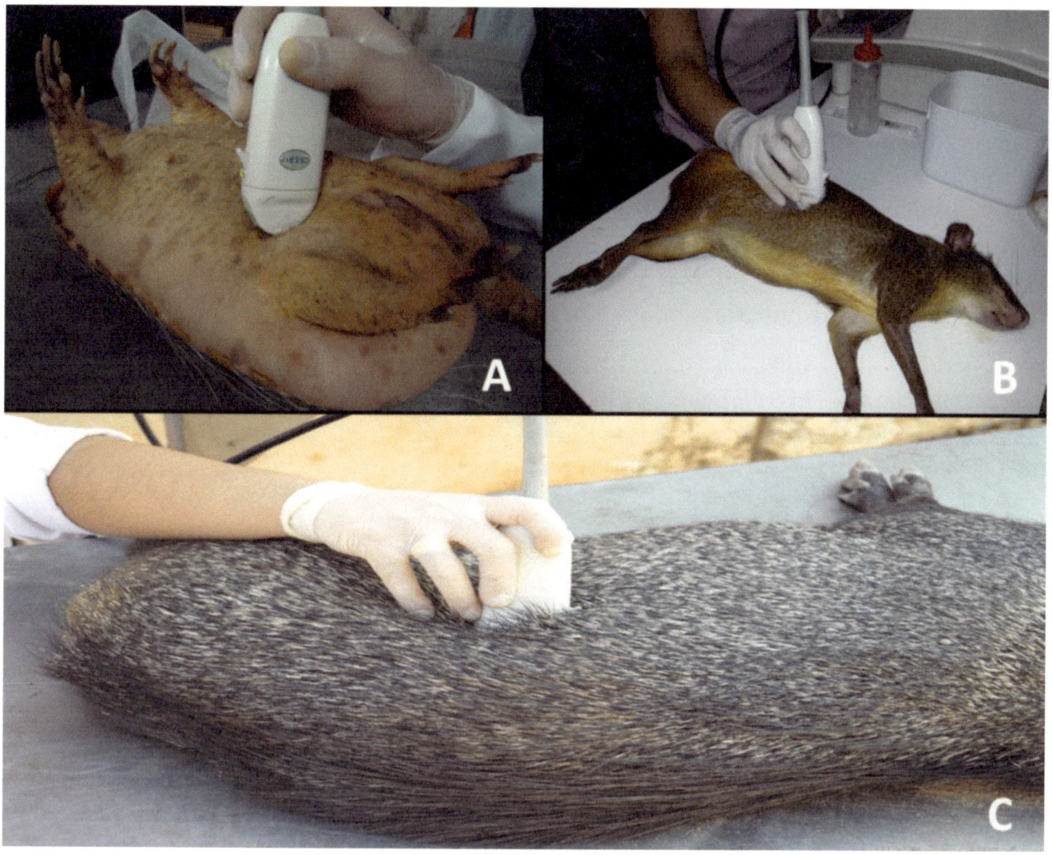

Figure 2. Placement of the ultrasound transducer for ovary monitoring in armadillo (A), agouti (B), and collared peccary (C).

follicles <4 mm increased and the number follicles ≥4 mm decreased in the same proportion. Additionally, the dominant follicle was defined as a follicle that attained a diameter ≥8 mm, and these findings provide rationale for the hypothesis that the increase in follicular size was associated with an increase in estradiol concentration. After ovulation, the corpus luteum was observed at the same location within the next 3 days [84].

For wood bison (*Bison bison athabascae*), the ultrasound was used for transvaginal ultrasound-guided follicular aspiration after an effective superovulatory protocol (association of PGF, eCG, and FSH). Numerous follicles ≥5 mm were easily detected on day 14 after treatment, featuring the technique as effective [89].

Transrectal ultrasound (4–7 MHz) exams were performed to follow the appearance of ovarian follicles after different synchronization protocols in the Przewalski's horse (*Equus ferus przewalskii*). The characterization of ovarian structures, that is, numbers of follicle, follicle size, and the presence of a corpus luteum, was easily performed [90].

The use of ultrasound in African elephants has been well characterized. It has proven to be a valuable tool for use with ARTs and has enormous potential for evaluating the efficiency of hormonal therapies used to treat reproductive dysfunction. Transrectal ultrasound showed that this species presents a peculiar pattern of follicular development in the ovary, associated with two LH surges: the first with formation of multiple small follicles and the second with a single large ovulatory follicle [91].

In order to determine the ideal day for artificial insemination in white rhinoceros, the ovarian follicle sizes were visualized by ultrasound. After measurement of preovulatory follicle (mean 2.7 cm), ovulation was induced with GnRH analog administration. The artificial insemination procedure resulted in two pregnancies. In addition, ultrasound documented the postpartum involution of the uterus, complete reabsorption of accumulated intrauterine fluid, and the development of a preovulatory follicle 30 days postpartum [14].

Many studies using ultrasonography have been described for estrus monitoring [34] and synchronization [92] in collared peccaries. Ovarian follicles measuring 0.2 ± 0.1 cm were visualized during the estrogen peak; corpora lutea, presented as hyperechoic regions measuring 0.4 ± 0.2 cm, were identified during luteal phase [34].

Regarding carnivores, the ultrasound was useful to characterize the ovaries of maned wolf (*C. brachyurus*) in captivity. In this species, the description of the ovaries (mean 1.02 cm length and 0.67 cm width) and follicles (mean 1.12 cm length and 0.32 cm width) is similar to that reported for domestic bitches [93].

The lynx (*Lynx* sp.), a most critically endangered felid, presents unique reproductive strategy with a monoestrus cycle persisting corpora lutea over the years. Painer et al. [94] evaluated whether artificial luteolysis could be achieved with common luteolytic drugs and if luteolysis would induce a subsequent natural estrus. In this case, the ultrasound was used as a primordial method for the identification of nonstructural regression of corpora lutea and subsequent spontaneous estrus induction after treatment with PGF2α analog (cloprostenol, 2.5 mg/kg).

However, in the marsupial wombat (*L. latifrons*), because of the opacity of the ovarian bursa, the transabdominal ultrasonography was unsuccessful for confirming ovulation, detecting the number of follicles in stimulated ovaries or the presence of the preovulatory follicle [95].

Recently, the monitoring of reproductive physiology in a Xenarthra, the six-banded armadillo, was made possible by ultrasound screening of the ovary. Using a microconvex transducer (8.0 MHz), it was possible to detect the ovary in 88.3% of the attempts, with defined structures, rounded and slightly hypoechoic compared to adjacent tissue [37]. The same study showed that, in 52% of the monitored ovaries in the follicular phase, it was possible to identify the presence of growing ovarian follicles, measuring on average $0.2 \pm 0.1 \times 0.2 \pm 0.2$ cm. In addition, during the luteal phase, the corpus luteum was observed in 60% of the ovaries, ranging from 0.1 to 0.2 cm [37].

Regarding rodents, a study carried out in red-rumped agoutis used different techniques to monitor the estrus cycle, including the ultrasound. Although it failed to differentiate the ovarian morphology during the different phases of the estrus cycle, the ultrasound was efficient to identify and measure follicles during the follicular phase, with an average diameter of 1 ± 0.5 mm; conversely, only in 12.5% of luteal phase, corpora lutea measuring 1.4 ± 0.9 mm were identified. Authors related the difficulty in identifying the ovary to its reduced size, as well as to the presence of adjacent fat [43].

6. Other possibilities

Thermography is a modern, noninvasive, and safe technique that measures the temperature in a surface based on its infrared radiation emission, given that the superficial heating of an animal is influenced by local circulation and tissue metabolism, which are generally constant [96]. Areas with higher metabolic rates show a higher temperature than areas with less tissue activity; therefore, surface temperature changes are caused by changes in local perfusion [97]. The increased local blood flow is linked to the rising of plasma estrogens, reflected by vulvar reddening and swelling that have been widely reported as typical estrus signs [98]. Altogether, infrared thermography has the potential to evaluate these physiological changes by monitoring the increase of temperature on the vulvar skin, with the objective of establishing a relationship between vulvar temperature fluctuation and ovulation [99].

Unfortunately, thermography has some limitations: good quality thermo-cameras can be very expensive, and also the maintenance of the camera can be expensive [97]; care must be taken when getting images in sunlight or in high humidity conditions, also with convective heat loss due to wind or when surfaces are dirty. Radiation measured by the camera does not only depend upon the temperature of the object but is also a function of its emissivity and conductivity [100]. Infrared thermography has proved to be highly sensitive to changes in the environmental conditions. Factors such as air flow, moisture, fluctuations in the environmental temperature, level of physical activity, and animal's stance before the measurement can induce a considerable variation in these readings, which may limit the applicability of this technology under field conditions, where these factors are difficult to control [99].

Currently, thermography is being used in some domestic species for estrus cycle monitoring as bovine [96, 99], swine [101], and equine [102]. In wild animals, this technique is still underused; however, it is noteworthy that, in addition to its other advantages, this is a noninvasive technique, which in certain conditions may be very useful, to avoid the immobilization of the animal [103]. Sykes et al. [104] defend that infrared thermography could be valuable for estrus detection in zoological species due to the possibility of observing and monitoring the animals in a natural environment with little human interference. However, variation among species could hinder the accurate estrus detection in all species. Difference in the length of estrus cycle and in the temperature gradients of the vulva also needs to be mapped out over continuous cycles to assess uniformity. In this context, continuous research is needed for both domestic and zoological species to validate thermography as a reliable tool for estrus detection.

In dealing with wildlife management, the preferential use of less or noninvasive techniques is required since this is necessary for maintaining the physiological behavior of the animals and reducing stressful situations. Therefore, several modern and practical methods having the potential to be adapted from domestic to wild animals have been developed, such as the use of pedometers, video cameras, and electronic odor detector, among others.

Pedometer is a real-time watch used for time interval measuring of the animal activity [100]. This activity measurer is commonly used at the neck or legs in cows, being connected to a computerized receiver for movement analysis. Some pedometer emits signals in a form of light when cows show increased activity. It is observed that cows in heat are more mobile and walk two to four times more when compared to non-estrus animals. Data of cow activity recoded with the help of pedometer has good correlation with estrus, thus resulting in a heat detection efficiency from 90 to 96%. Its main limitations are the high cost for acquisition and replacement of lost equipment [105].

The principle of the electronic odor detector is based on the detection of sex pheromones related to heat. The pheromones are the natural olfactory signal for male that cow emits during estrus. It is up to 90% efficient. Even if the project is running for a successful future, further development steps are anticipated [106].

6.1. General considerations

The development of reliable and less-invasive techniques for monitoring the reproductive cycle of wild mammals is required to optimize the captive breeding management. These techniques are needed for the use of reproductive biotechnologies applied for either preservation or production. Understanding the changes in reproductive behavior of wild animals is therefore critical to better estrus monitoring—which allows the application of reproductive biotechnologies—as well as improving the management of these animals [11, 107]. Therefore, the use of noninvasive techniques to monitor the reproductive status is of paramount importance to avoid stress and its induced changes in physiology.

Author details

Alexandre R. Silva[1]*, Nei Moreira[2], Alexsandra F. Pereira[3], Gislayne C.X. Peixoto[1], Keilla M. Maia[1], Lívia B. Campos[1] and Alana A. Borges[3]

*Address all correspondence to: legio2000@yahoo.com

1 Laboratory of Animal Germplasm Conservation, UFERSA, Mossoró, RN, Brazil

2 Department of Biosciences, UFPR, Palotina, PR, Brazil

3 Laboratory of Animal Biotechnology, UFERSA, Mossoró, RN, Brazil

References

[1] Guimarães MABV. A aplicação de técnicas de reprodução assistida em animais silvestres mantidos em cativeiro [The application of assisted reproduction techniques to wild animals kept in captivity]. Revista Brasileira de Reprodução Animal. 2001;**25**:116-117

[2] Clay AM, Estes RD, Thompson KV, Wildt DE, Monfort SL. Endocrine patterns of the estrous cycle and pregnancy of wildebeest in the Serengeti ecosystem. General and Comparative Endocrinology. 2010;**166**:365-371

[3] Lees CM, Wilcken J. Sustaining the Ark: The challenges faced by zoos in maintaining viable populations. International Zoo Yearbook. 2009;**43**:6-18

[4] Abáigar T, Domenéa MA, Cassinello J. Characterization of the estrous cycle and reproductive traits of the aoudad (*Ammotragus lervia*) in captivity. Theriogenology. 2012;**77**:1759-1766

[5] Godde S, Humbert L, Cote SD, Reale D, Whitehead H. Correcting for the impact of gregariousness in social network analyses. Animal Behaviour. 2013;**85**:553-558

[6] SankarGanesh D, Ramachandran R, Muniasamy S, Saravanakumar VR, Suriyakala U, Kannan S, Archunan G, Achiraman S. A correlation of fecal volatiles and steroid hormone profiles with behavioral expression during estrous cycle of goat, *Capra hircus*. General and Comparative Endocrinology. 2014;**206**:178-183

[7] Mainguy J, Côté SD, Cardinal E, Houle M. Mating tactics and mate choice in relation to age and social rank in male mountain goats. Journal Mammalogy. 2008;**89**:626-635

[8] Khonmee J, Brown JL, Taya K, Rojanasthien S, Punyapornwithaya V, Thumasanukul D, Kongphoemphun A, Siriaroonrat B, Tipkantha W, Pongpiachan P, Thitaram C. Assessment of ovarian activity in captive goral (*Naemorhedus griseus*) using noninvasive fecal steroid monitoring. Theriogenology. 2014;**82**:997-1006

[9] Silva SSB, Le Pendu Y, Ohashi OM, Oba E, Albuquerque NI, Garcia AR, Mayor P, Guimarães DAA. Sexual behavior of *Pecari tajacu* (Cetartiodactyla: Tayassuidae) during periovulatory and early gestation periods. Behavioural Processes. 2016;**131**:68-73

[10] Ghosal R, Kalaivanan N, Sukumar R, Seshagiri PB. Assessment of estrus cyclicity in the Asian elephant (*Elephas maximus*) by measurement of fecal progesterone metabolite 5a-P-3OH, using a non-invasive assay. General and Comparative Endocrinology. 2012;**175**:100-108

[11] Glaeser SS, Hunt KE, Martin MS, Finnegan M, Brown JL. Investigation of individual and group variability in estrous cycle characteristics in female Asian elephants (*Elephas maximus*) at the Oregon Zoo. Theriogenology. 2012;**78**:285-296

[12] Vidya TNC, Sukumar R. Social and reproductive behaviour in elephants. Current Science. 2005;**89**:1200-1207

[13] Santiago-Moreno J, Gómez-Brunet A, Toledano-Díaz A, Pulido-Pastor A, López-Sebastián A. Social dominance and breeding activity in Spanish ibex (*Capra pyrenaica*) maintained in captivity. Reproduction Fertility and Development. 2007;**19**:436-442

[14] Hildebrandt TB, Hermes R, Walzer C, Sós E, Molnar V, Mezösi L, Schnorrenberg A, Silinski S, Streich J, Schwarzenberger F, Göritz F. Artificial insemination in the anoestrous and the postpartum white rhinoceros using GnRH analogue to induce ovulation. Theriogenology. 2007;**67**:1473-1484

[15] Umapathy G, Sontakke SD, Srinivasu K, Kiran T, Kholkute SD, Shivaji S. Estrus behavior and fecal steroid profiles in the Asiatic lion (*Panthera leo persica*) during natural and gonadotropin-induced estrus. Animal Reproduction Science. 2007;**101**:313-325

[16] Frederick C, Kyes R, Hunt K, Collins D, Durrant B, Wasser SK. Methods of estrus detection and correlates of the reproductive cycle in the sun bear (*Helarctos malayanus*). Theriogenology. 2010;**74**:1121-1135

[17] North LA, Harder JD. Characterization of the estrous cycle and assessment of reproductive status in Matschie's tree kangaroo (*Dendrolagus matschiei*) with fecal progestin profiles. General and Comparative Endocrinology. 2008;**156**:173-180

[18] Reddy KCS, Raju KGS, Rao KS, Rao KBR. Vaginal cytology, vaginoscopy and progesterone profile: Breeding tools in bitches. Iraqi Journal of Veterinary Science. 2011;**25**:51-54

[19] Jainudeen MR, Eisenberg JF, Tilakeratne N. Oestrous cycle of the Asiatic elephant, *Elephas maximus*, in captivity. Journal of Reproduction and Fertility. 1971;**27**:321-328

[20] Watson PF, D'Souza FD. Detection of oestrus in the African elephant (*Loxodonta africana*). Theriogenology. 1975;**4**:203-209

[21] Doi O, Komatsumoto M, Terazono M, Wada S, Akihisa N, Sakamoto H, Hamasaki T, Yanagimoto H, Nakano K, Matsuoka K, Ito A, Kusunoki A, Nakamura T. Exfoliative cytology in vaginal vestibule of female Asian elephants: Relation to circulating progesterone concentrations. Zoological Science. 2000;**17**:1303-1309

[22] Payne KB, Langbauer WR, Thomas EM. Infrasonic calls of the Asian elephant (*Elephas maximus*). Behavioral Ecology and Sociobiology. 1986;**18**:297-301

[23] Poole JH. Mate guarding, reproductive success and female choice in African elephants. Animal Behavior. 1989;**37**:842-849

[24] Bittencourt VL, De Paula TAR, Costa MELT, Malta MCC, Bastos JAB. Acompanhamento do ciclo reprodutivo de lobo guará (*Chrysocion brachyurus*) adulta através de citologia vaginal. In: Proceedings of the Encontro da Associação Brasileira de Veterinários de Animais Selvagens; ABRAVAS: Vitória, Espirito Santo; 2002

[25] Weinhardt D, Rodden M. Management of reproduction. In: Fletchall NB, Rodden M, Taylor S. Husbandry Manual for the Maned Wolf (*Chrysocyon brachyurus*). Washington; 1995;29-31. (http://www.zoocentral.dk/uploads/4/9/7/5/49755431/wolf_maned_-_aza_-_1995.pdf)

[26] Seal US, Tilson RL, Plotka ED, Reindl NJ, Seal MF. Behavioral indicators and endocrine correlates of estrous and anestrous in Siberian tigers. In: Tilson RL, Seal US. In Tigers of the World: The Biology, Biopolitics, Management, and Conservation of an Endangered Species. Park Ridge, NJ: Noyes Publications; 1987. pp. 244-254

[27] Brown JL, Wasser SK, Wildt DE, Graham LH. Comparative aspects of steroid hormone metabolism and ovarian activity in felids, measured noninvasively in feces. Biology of Reproduction. 1994;**51**:776-786

[28] Moreira N, Monteiro-Filho EL, Moraes W, Swanson WF, Graham LH, Pasquali OL, Gomes ML, Morais RN, Wildt DE, Brown JL. Reproductive steroid hormones and ovarian activity in felids of the *Leopardus* Genus. Zoo Biology. 2001;**20**:103-116

[29] Silva GCO, Berbare PEB, Zaccariotti RL, Corrêa SHR, Oliveira CA, Guimarães MABV. Estudo da correlação das características citológicas vaginais e os níveis séricos de estradiol e progesterona em leão africano (*Panthera leo*) mantidos em cativeiro. Brazilian Journal of Veterinary Research and Animal Science. 2006;**43**:227-232

[30] Asa CS, Junge RE, Bircher JS, Noble GA, Sarri KJ, Plotka ED. Assessing reproductive cycles and pregnancy in cheetahs (*Acinonyx jubatus*) by vaginal cytology. Zoo Biology. 1992;**11**:139-151

[31] Bonney RC, Moore HDM, Jones DM. Plasma concentrations of oestradiol-17β and progesterone, and laparoscopic observations of the ovary in the puma (*Felis concolor*) during oestrus, pseudopregnancy and pregnancy. Journal of Reproduction and Fertility. 1981;**63**:523-532

[32] Paz RCR, Adania CH, Barnabe VH, Barnabe RC. Vaginal cytology for estrus detection in ocelot (*Leopardus pardalis*). Arquivo Brasileiro Medicina Veterinária Zootecnia. 2010;**62**:1409-1414

[33] Fredericka C, Kyesb C, Huntc K, Collinsd D, Durrante B, Wasserf SK. Methods of estrus detection and correlates of the reproductive cycle in the sun bear (*Helarctos malayanus*). Theriogenology. 2010;**74**:1121-1135

[34] Maia KM, Peixoto GCX, Campos LB, Bezerra JAB, Ricarte, ARF, Moreira N, Oliveira MF, Silva AR. Estrus cycle monitoring of captive collared peccaries (*Pecari tajacu*) in semiarid conditions. Pesquisa Veterinária Brasileira. 2014;**34**:1115-1120

[35] Guimarães DA, Garcia SCG, Pendu Y, Albuquerque NI. Determinação do ciclo estral em catetos *Pecari tajacu*: Aspectos colpocitológicos e clínicos. Acta Amazônica. 2011;**41**:583-588

[36] Snoeck PPN, Cruz ACB, Catenacci LS, Cassano CR. Vaginal cytology of maned sloth (*Bradypus torquatus*). Pesquisa Veterinária Brasileira. 2011;**31**:271-275

[37] Campos LB, Peixoto GCX, Lima GL, Castelo TS, Silva AM, Freitas CIA, Silva, AR. Monitoring the reproductive physiology of six-banded armadillos (*Euphractus sexcinctus*, Linnaeus, 1758) through different techniques. Reproduction in Domestic Animals. 2016;**51**:736-742

[38] Kusuda S, Endoh T, Tanaka H, Adachi I, Doi O, Kimura J. Relationship between gonadal steroid hormones and vulvar bleeding in southern tamandua, *Tamandua tetradactyla*. Zoo Biology. 2011;**30**:212-217

[39] Costa TO, Fernandes WOB, Costa CLC, Maia RM, Viana ARS, Freitas CIA. Aspectos reprodutivos em fêmeas de tatu-peba (Euphractus sexcinctus) mantidas em cativeiro. Acta Veterinaria Brasilica. 2014;**8**:27

[40] Felipe AE, Cabodevila J, Callejas S. Characterization of the estrous cycle of the *Myocastor coypus* (coypu) by means of exfoliative colpocytology. Mastozoología Neotropical/ Journal of Neotropical Mammalogy. 2001;**8**:129-137

[41] Busso JM, Florit E, Ponzio MF, Fiol de Cuneo M, Ruiz RD. Identificación de la "ventana de fertilidad" mediante monitoreo estral no invasivo en chinchilla. [Noninvasive monitoring of estral cycles in chinchilla: Identification of fertile periods]. In: Proceedings of the XXII Congreso Latinoamericano y 1er Iberoamericano de Ciencias Fisiológicas. Sociedad Argentina de Fisiologia: Buenos Aires; 2006

[42] Guimarães, DA, Bastos LV, Ferreira ACS, Luz-Ramos RS, Ohashi OM, Ribeiro HL. Características reprodutivas da paca fêmea (*Agouti paca*) criada em cativeiro. Acta Amazônica. 2008;**38**:531-538

[43] Weir B. Some observations on reproduction in the female agouti (*Dasyprocta agouti*). Journal of Reproduction and Fertility. 1971;**24**:203-211

[44] Prendergast BJ, Zucker I, Nelson RJ. Mammalian seasonal rhythms: Behavior and neuroendocrine substrates. In: Pfaff DW, Arnold AP, Etgen AM, Fahrbach SE, Rubin RT. Hormones, Brain and Behavior. San Diego, CA: Academic Press; 2002. 93-156

[45] Weir B. Reproductive characteristics of hystricomorph rodents. Symposia of the Zoological Society of London. 1974;**34**:265-301

[46] Hunter RHF, Hunt DM, Chang MC. Temporal and cytological aspects of fertilization and early development in the guinea pig, *Cavia porcellus*. The Anatomical Record. 1969;**165**:411-430

[47] Kleiman D. Reproduction in the female green Acouchi, *Myoprocta pratti* Pocock. Journal of Reproduction and Fertility. 1970;**23**:55-65

[48] Weir BJ. In: Hafez ESE, editors. Reproduction and Breeding Techniques for Laboratory Animals. Chinchilla: Lea and Febiger; 1970. 209-223

[49] Santos AC, Viana DC, Oliveira GB, Silva RS, Oliveira MF, Assis-Neto AC. Follicular development and morphological changes in the vaginal epithelium during the estrous cycle of *Galea spixii*. Microscopy Research and Technique. 2016;**80**:167-176

[50] West M, Galloway D, Shaw J, Tounson A, Paris MCJ. Oestrous cycle of the common wombat, *Vombatus ursinus*, in Victoria, Australia. Reproduction Fertility and Development. 2004;**16**:339-346

[51] Finlayson GR, Shimmin GA, Taggart DA, Skinner JF, Gilmore A, Paris MCJ. Oestrous cycle of captive southern hairy-nosed wombats (*Lasiorhinus latifrons*) in South Australia, Australia. Animal Reproduction Science. 2006;**95**:295-306

[52] MacCallum CA. The reproductive biology of the common wombat (*Vombatus ursinus*): Studies towards the development of an artificial insemination protocol. Faculty of Science (School of Animal Studies) [Master's thesis]. Gatton: The University of Queensland; 2004

[53] West M. The oestrous cycle and manipulation of reproduction in the common wombat (*Vombatus ursinus*). Reproductive Sciences [PhD thesis]: Monash University, Melbourne; 2002

[54] Hogan LA, Phillips CJC, Lisle A, Keeley T, Horsup AB, Janssen T, Johnston SD. Non-invasive methods of oestrus detection in captive Southern hairy-nosed wombats (*Lasiorhinus latifrons*). Animal Reproduction Science. 2010;**119**:293-304

[55] Peters DG, Rose RW. The oestrus cycle and basal body temperature in the common wombat (*Vombatus ursinus*). Journal of Reproduction and Fertility. 1979;**57**:453-460

http://dx.doi.org/10.5772/intechopen.69444

[56] Hogan LA, Phillips CJC, Lisle A, Horsup AB, Janssen T, Johnston SD. Reproductive behaviour of the Southern hairy-nosed wombat (*Lasiorhinus latifrons*). Australian Journal of Zoology. 2010b;**58**:350-361

[57] Hogan LA, Janssen T, Johnston SD. Wombat reproduction (Marsupialia; Vombatidae): An update and future directions for the development of artificial breeding technology. Reproduction. 2013;**145**:R157-R173

[58] Schwarzenberger F, Brown JL. Hormone monitoring: An important tool for the breeding management of wildlife species. Veterinary Medicine Austria. 2013;**100**:209-225

[59] Singh MD, Morris, MJ, Guimarães DA, Bourne G, Garcia GW. Serological evaluation of ovarian steroids of red-rumped agouti (*Dasyprocta leporina*) during the estrous cycle phases. Animal Reproduction Science. 2016;**175**:27-32

[60] Steinman KJ, O'Brien JK, Monfort SL, Robeck TR. Characterization of the estrous cycle in female beluga (*Delphinapterus leucas*) using urinary endocrine monitoring and transabdominal ultrasound: Evidence of facultative induced ovulation. General and Comparative Endocrinology. 2012;**175**:389-397

[61] Illera JC, Silván G, Cáceres S, Carbonell MD, Gerique C, Martínez-Fernández L, Munro C, Casares M. Assessment of ovarian cycles in the African elephant (*Loxodonta africana*) by measurement of salivary progesterone metabolites. Zoo Biology. 2014;**33**:245-249

[62] Terwissen CV, Mastromonaco GF, Murray DL. Enzyme immunoassays as a method for quantifying hair reproductive hormones in two felid species. Conservation Physiology. 2014;**2**:cou044-cou053

[63] Heistermann M. Non-invasive monitoring of endocrine status in laboratory primates: Methods, guidelines and applications. Advances in Science and Research. 2010;**5**:1-9

[64] Kersey DC, Dehnhard M. The use of noninvasive and minimally invasive methods in endocrinology for threatened mammalian species conservation. General and Comparative Endocrinology. 2014;**203**:296-306

[65] Habumuremyi S, Stephens C, Fawcett KA, Deschner T, Robbins M. Endocrine assessment of ovarian cycle activity in wild female mountain gorillas (*Gorilla beringei beringei*). Physiology & Behavior. 2016;**157**:185-195

[66] Mithileshwari C, Srivastava T, Kumar V, Kumar A, Umapathy G. Non-invasive assessment of fecal progestagens and pregnancy detection in Himalayan musk deer (*Moschus chrysogaster*). Theriogenology. 2016;**85**:216-223

[67] Schwarzenberger F, Rietschel W, Vahala J, Holeckova D, Thomas P, Maltzan J, Baumgartner K, Schaftenaar W. Fecal progesterone, estrogen, and androgen metabolites for noninvasive monitoring of reproductive function in the female Indian rhinoceros, *Rhinoceros unicornis*. General and Comparative Endocrinology. 2000;**119**:300-307

[68] Stoops MA, MacKinnon KM, Roth TL. Longitudinal fecal hormone analysis for monitoring reproductive activity in the female polar bear (*Ursus maritimus*). Theriogenology. 2012;**78**:1977-1986

[69] Lasley B. Endocrine research advances in breeding endangered species. International Zoo Yearbook. 1980;**20**:166-170

[70] Schwarzenberger F, Möstl E, Palme R, Bamberg E. Faecal steroid analysis for non-invasive monitoring of reproductive status in farm, wild and zoo animals. Animal Reproduction Science. 1996;**42**:515-526

[71] Muren, Kusuda S, Doi O, Naito H, Hashikawa H. Puberty, ovarian cycle, pregnancy, and postpartum ovulation in captive Sichuan golden monkeys (*Rhinopithecus roxellana*) based on changes in urinary and fecal gonadal steroid metabolites. Theriogenology. 2016;**87**:179-186

[72] Kusuda S, Adachi I, Fujioka K, Nakamura M, Amano-Hanzawa N, Goto N, Furuhashia S, Doi O. Reproductive characteristics of female lesser mouse deer (*Tragulus javanicus*) based on fecal progestagens and breeding records. Animal Reproduction Science. 2013;**137**:69-73

[73] Palme R, Möstl E. Biotin-streptavidin enzyme immunoassay for the determination of oestrogens and androgens in boar faeces. Advances of Steroid Analysis. 1994;**93**:111-117

[74] Niemuller CA, Shaw HJ, Hodges JK. Non-invasive monitoring of ovarian function in Asian elephants (*Elephas maximus*) by measurement of urinary 5β-pregnanetriol. Journal of Reproduction and Fertility. 1993;**99**:617-625

[75] Amaral RS, Rosas FC, Silva VM, Nichi M, Oliveira CA. Endocrine monitoring of the ovarian cycle in captive female Amazonian manatees (*Trichechus inunguis*). Animal Reproduction Science. 2013;**142**:84-88

[76] Kapoor A, Lubach G, Hedman C, Ziegler TE, Coe CL. Hormones in infant rhesus monkeys (*Macaca mulatta*) hair at birth provide a window into the fetal environment. Pediatric Research. 2014;**75**:476-481

[77] Patzl M, Schwarzenberger F, Osmann C, Bamberg E, Bartmann W. Monitoring ovarian cycle and pregnancy in the giant anteater (*Myrmecophaga tridactyla*) by faecal progestagen and oestrogen analysis. Animal Reproduction Science. 1998;**53**:209-219

[78] Schwarzenberger F, Walzer C, Tomasova K, Vahala J, Meister J, Goodrowe KL, Zima J, Strauss F, Lynch M. Fecal progesterone metabolite analysis for non-invasive monitoring of reproductive function in the white rhinoceros (*Ceratotherium simum*). Animal Reproduction Science. 1998;**53**:173-190

[79] MacKinnon KM, Guilfoyle MJ, Swanson WF, Stoops MA. Assessment of the reproductive physiology of the potto (*Perodicticus potto*) through fecal hormone metabolite analyses and trans-abdominal ultrasonography. Zoo Biology. 2015;**34**:244-254

[80] Robeck TR, Steinman KJ, Yoshioka M, Jensen E, O'Brien JK, Katsumata E, Gili C, McBain JF, Sweeney J, Monfort SL. Estrous cycle characterization and artificial insemination using frozen-thawed spermatozoa in the bottlenose dolphin (*Tursiops truncatus*). Reproduction. 2005;**129**:659-674

[81] Robeck TR, Steinman KJ, Greenwell M, Ramirez K, Van Bonn W, Yoshioka M, Katsumata E, Dalton L, Osborn S, O'Brien JK. Seasonality, estrous cycle characterization, estrus synchronization, semen cryopreservation, and artificial insemination in the Pacific white-sided dolphin (*Lagenorhynchus obliquidens*). Reproduction. 2009;**138**:391-405

[82] Ma ZF. Studies on Disciplinary of Ovarian Activities in the Northeast Sika Deer Within-Estrous Cycle. Journal of Northeast Agricultural University; 2007. pp. 60-68

[83] Mattle FME, Pryce CR, Anzenberger G. Different ovarian responses to potential mates underlie species-specific breeding strategies in common marmoset and Goeldi's monkey. Hormones and Behavior. 2008;**54**:302-311

[84] Chen XM, Wei HJ, Yang YF, Xue HL, Zhao WG, Zhao M. Serum hormone concentrations and ovarian follicular wave emergence in Jilin sika deer (*Cervus nippon hortulorum*) after synchronization of estrous cycles. Animal Reproduction Science. 2015;**153**:44-49

[85] Oerke AK, Einspanier A, Hodges JK. Noninvasive monitoring of follicle development, ovulation, and corpus luteum formation in the marmoset monkey (*Callithrix jacchus*) by ultrasonography. American Journal of Primatology. 1996;**39**:99-113

[86] Domingues SFS, Caldas-Bussiere MC, Martins ND, Mattos MRF, Simões-Mattos L. A fêmea de Macaco-prego (*Cebus apella* Linnaeus, 1758). Revista Ciência Agrarias Suplemento. 2005;**43**:1-9

[87] Ortiz RE, Ortiz AC, Gajardo G, Zepeda AJ, Parraguez VH, Ortiz ME, Croxato HB. Cytologic, hormonal, and ultrasonographic correlates of the menstrual cycle of the new world monkey *Cebus apella*. American Journal of Primatology. 2005;**66**:233-244

[88] McCorkell RB, Woodbury MR, Adams GP. Evaluation of an ovarian synchronization scheme for fixed-time artificial insemination in wapiti. Theriogenology. 2007;**67**:1217-1223

[89] Palomino JM, McCorkell RB, Woodbury MR, Cervantes MP, Adams GP. Ovarian superstimulation and oocyte collection in wood bison (*Bison bison athabascae*) during the ovulatory season. Theriogenology. 2014;**81**:250-256

[90] Collins CW, Monfort SL, Vick MM, Wolfe BA, Weiss RB, Keefer CL, Songsasen N. Oral and injectable synthetic progestagens effectively manipulate the estrous cycle in the Przewalski's horse (*Equus ferus przewalskii*). Animal Reproduction Science. 2014;**148**:42-52

[91] Hermes R, Olson D, Goritz F, Brown JL, Schmitt DL, Hagan D, Peterson JS, Fritsch G. *Loxodonta africana* Hildebrandt TB. Ultrasonography of the estrous cycle in female African elephants. Zoo Biology. 2000;**19**:369-382

[92] Peixoto GCX. Aplicação de biotécnicas para monitoramento e controle do ciclo estralde espécies silvestres do bioma Caatinga [PhD thesis]. Programa de Pós-Graduação em Biotecnologia da Rede Nordeste de Biotecnologia (RENORBIO), Natal; 2016

[93] Guimarães LD, Hage MCFNS, Paula TAR, Borges APB, Carretta Junior M, Oliveira AR, Carneiro FT, Silva VHD. Abdominal and pelvic ultrasound study of the maned Wolf (*Chrysocyon brachyurus*). Pesquisa Veterinária Brasileira. 2013;**33**:265-272

[94] Painer J, Goeritz F, Dehnhard M, Hildebrandt TB, Naidenko SV, Sánchez I, Muñoz MAQ, Jewgenow K. Hormone-induced luteolysis on physiologically persisting corpora lutea in Eurasian and Iberian lynx (*Lynx lynx* and *Lynx pardinus*). Theriogenology. 2014;**82**:557-562

[95] Druery GV, Rival MD, Taggart DA, Shimmin GA, Horsup AB, Temple-Smith PD, Paris DB, Paris MCJ. Timing of ovulation in the gonadotrophin-stimulated southern hairy-nosed wombat, *Lasiorhinus latifrons*. Reproduction, Fertility and Development. 2005;**17**:246

[96] Metzner M, Sauter-Louis C, Seemueller A, Petzl W, Klee W. Infrared thermography of the udder surface of dairy cattle: Characteristics, methods, and correlation with rectal temperature. The Veterinary Journal. 2014;**199**:57-62

[97] Redaelli V, Bergero D, Zucca E, Ferrucci F, Costa LN, Crosta L, Luzi F. Use of thermography techniques in equines: Principles and applications. Journal of Equine Veterinary Science. 2014;**34**:345-350

[98] Langendijk P, Van den Brand H, Soede NM, Kemp B. Effect of boar contact on follicular development and on estrus expression after weaning in primiparous sows. Theriogenology. 2000;**54**:1295-1303

[99] Simões VG, Lyazrhi F, Picard-Hagen N, Gayrard V, Martineau GP, WaretSzkuta A. Variations in the vulvar temperature of sows during proestrus and estrus as determined by infrared thermography and its relation to ovulation. Theriogenology. 2014;**82**:1080-1085

[100] Knízková I, Kunc P, Gürdíl GAK, Pinar Y, Selví KÇ. Applications of infrared thermography in animal production. Journal of the Faculty of Agriculture. 2007;**22**:329-336

[101] Luño V, Gil L, Jerez RA, Malo C, González N, Grandía J. Determination of ovulation time in sows based on skin temperature and genital electrical resistance changes. Veterinary Record. 2013;**172**:579

[102] Stelletta C, Gianesella M, Vencato J, Fiore E, Morgante M. Thermographic applications in Veterinary Medicine. In: Prakash RV. Infrared Thermography. Rijeka: InTech; 2012. pp. 117-140

[103] Durrant BS, Ravida N, Spady T, Cheng A. New technologies for the study of carnivore reproduction. Theriogenology. 2006;**66**:1729-1736

[104] Sykes DJ, Couvillion JS, Cromiak A, Bowers S, Schenck E, Crenshaw M, Ryan PL. The use of digital infrared thermal imaging to detect estrus in gilts. Theriogenology. 2012;**78**:147-152

[105] Brehme U, Stollberh U, Holz R, Schleusenner T. ALT pedometer—New sensor aided measurement system for improvement in oestrus detection. Electronics in Agriculture. 2008;**62**:73-80

[106] Weigerinck W, Setkus A, Buda, V, Borg-Karlson AK, Mozuraitis R, de Gee A. Bovinose: Pheromone-based sensor system for detecting estrus in dairy cows. Procedia Computer Science. 2011;**7**:340342

[107] Archunan G, Rajagopal T. Detection of estrus in Indian blackbuck: Behavioural, hormonal and urinary volatiles evaluation. General and Comparative Endocrinology. 2013;**181**:156-166

Chapter 3

Markers for Sperm Freezability and Relevance of Transcriptome Studies in Semen Cryopreservation: A Review

Leyland Fraser

Additional information is available at the end of the chapter

http://dx.doi.org/10.5772/intechopen.68651

Abstract

Advances in sperm assessment techniques have offered new perspectives to improve the technology of semen cryopreservation. This review addresses some recent achievements in the proteomics of seminal plasma and spermatozoa and exemplifies its importance as markers for sperm fertility following cryopreservation. Recent advances in transcriptome studies on sperm RNA-Seq data have generated new information aimed to unravel the physiological roles of RNAs in the sperm-egg fertilization processes and their associations with male fertility. The relevance of the sperm freezability markers and the potential associations of RNA-profiling sequences with the sperm biological functions have been discussed.

Keywords: spermatozoa, frozen-thawed semen, RNA-Seq, bioinformatics studies

1. Introduction

Cryopreservation of semen allows the preservation of good genetic resources and the protection of endangered species [1–5]. While a great deal of efforts has been done over the last several years to improve the semen cryopreservation technology, effective cryosurvival of spermatozoa from various animal species, including the boar and stallion, still remains elusive and a cryobiological enigma [1]. Cryo-induced oxidative stress is associated with excess production of reactive oxygen species (ROS), resulting in biochemical and physical damage to the sperm membrane structures and subsequently leading to reduced fertilizing ability of spermatozoa [4–6]. In the artificial insemination (AI) industry, there is a need to optimize the selection strategy for individuals with good freezability, so as to incorporate this information in the breeding program to improve the fertility of post-thaw semen [2, 3, 7]. Moreover, selection of animals with good semen freezability for cryopreservation and AI is a crucial step to improve the fertility levels of frozen-thawed semen [9, 10]. Furthermore, in some animal species, despite satisfactory results of fertility in liquid-stored semen, frozen-thawed semen does not give acceptable fertility results in AI practice in the commercial industry [2, 3, 9].

Accumulating evidence has indicated that inherent male variability in semen freezability is one of the factors responsible for marked differences in the sperm cryosurvival [2, 5, 7–10]. With regard to boar semen, studies have reported that differences in sperm freezability might be due to a genetic origin [7, 8]. Even though the underlying mechanisms responsible for the genetic differences associated with poor or good semen freezability are yet unknown, it has been suggested that the identification of sperm freezability markers might be the most efficient approach to improve the technology of semen cryopreservation.

Recent technological advances have confirmed that the spermatozoon carries epigenetic factors that constitute their epigenome, such as proper packaging of the chromatin with protamines, modifications of histones, and a large population of messenger ribonucleic acid (mRNA) and microRNA (miRNA) transcripts [11–13]. The diversity of the RNA constellation in the seminal plasma (SP) and spermatozoa has been used as a pattern for the genomic analysis of semen quality characteristics, particularly for the estimation of the fertility potential of spermatozoa [12–17]. Moreover, high-throughput sequencing demonstrates that several stable full-length mRNA transcripts are useful markers for sperm functions in fresh and frozen-thawed semen [17]. It has been hypothesized that transcriptome analysis of sperm RNA-Sequencing (RNA-Seq) data is required to explore the potential links between semen freezability and the transcript profiles of spermatozoa [18–20]. This review discusses recent accomplishments in molecular markers for the assessment of post-thaw sperm quality and exemplifies the significant relevance of transcriptome profiling by RNA-Seq in semen cryopreservation.

2. Markers for sperm functions

2.1. Motility and motion characteristics

Subjective motility evaluation is one of the most commonly used parameters to determine the quality of frozen-thawed semen for AI. Even though post-thaw sperm motility is a good indicator of viability, it is not always an accurate fertility predictor of an AI-semen dose [9]. Evaluations of sperm motility characteristics have been improved by the incorporation of the computer-assisted semen analysis (CASA) system, which measures several motility and motion parameters of spermatozoa that are closely related to fertility compared with subjective motility measurements [21–24]. Besides motility analysis, studies have confirmed that the velocity parameters, such as velocity straight line (VSL), velocity curvilinear (VCL), and velocity average path (VAP), are associated with the fertilizing capacity of frozen-thawed spermatozoa [21, 24].

2.2. Membrane integrity

Spermatozoa comprise several compartments enclosed within the acrosome, plasma membrane, and mitochondrial membranes, which act as physiological barriers that must remain intact to permit cell viability, particularly after cryopreservation [1, 2, 6, 10]. In recent years, several fluorescent probes have shown that the cryopreservation process compromises the sperm plasma membrane integrity (PMI), resulting in reduced fertilizing capacity of post-thaw semen [3–5, 23–29]. Post-thaw sperm PMI has been assessed with different fluorescent membrane probes, such as the dual SYBR-14 and propidium iodide (PI) assay [25, 28] or membrane-permeable substrate carboxyfluorescein diacetate (CFDA), a nonspecific esterase substrate [24]. The chlortetracycline (CTC) fluorescence assay has been used to detect capacitation-like changes in frozen-thawed spermatozoa, which may compromise their fertilizing ability [6, 10, 22–24, 29]. Cryo-induced changes in the acrosome membrane integrity (AMI) have been monitored by specific Giemsa-staining technique [25] or with fluorescent dyes, such as fluorescein isothiocyanate (FITC)-conjugated PNA (peanut agglutinin) or conjugated PSA (*Pisum sativum* agglutinin), known as plant lectins, which bind to glycoproteins in the outer acrosomal membrane [4, 5, 26, 27]. Studies have shown that the utilization of a triple staining—SYBR-14, phycoerythrin-conjugated PNA (PE-PNA), and PI (SYBR-14/PE-PNA/PI)—to simultaneously evaluate the PMI and AMI of frozen-thawed bull spermatozoa can be used effectively to assess post-thaw semen viability [26–28]. In a recent study, it has been demonstrated that FITC-PSA/PI-staining protocol can detect marked deterioration in both the PMI and AMI in frozen-thawed bull spermatozoa [4]. Earlier changes in the membrane permeability of frozen-thawed spermatozoa have been monitored with the calcium-dependent binding of Annexin-V/FITC/PI [21, 24, 26] or YO-PRO-1 assay [23, 25, 28], which is an impermeable membrane probe. Moreover, triple staining with YO-PRO-1, ethidium homodimer (Eth), and SNARF-1 (YO-PRO-1/Eth/SNARF-1) has been shown to give similar results with respect to PMI assessment of frozen-thawed spermatozoa compared with the Annexin-V/FITC/PI assay [27, 28]. Kumar et al. [21] reported that there were marked differences in the percentages of frozen-thawed spermatozoa with apoptotic-like changes between fertile and sub-fertile bulls, being significantly higher in the latter. Moreover, there is accumulating evidence indicating that the cryopreservation procedure induces apoptotic-like features in bovine spermatozoa, which appeared as ordered events during the freezing-thawing process, such as reduced mitochondrial membrane potential (MMP), increased caspase activation, and modifications in membrane permeability [6, 21, 24, 27, 28, 30]. Additionally, post-thaw PMI has been assessed with the hypo-osmotic swelling (HOS) test, which evaluates the functional membrane integrity of the acrosome and tail regions when spermatozoa are exposed to hypo-osmotic conditions [22, 24, 29].

Cryopreservation affects the lipid composition and organization of the sperm plasma membranes, resulting in leakage of valuable intracellular enzymes, such as antioxidants [4], acrosin [31], aspartate aminotransferase (AspAT) [32], or energy substrates, such as adenosine triphosphate (ATP) [33], which ultimately lead to cell death. Another measure of membrane damage to frozen-thawed spermatozoa is the degree of lipid peroxidation (LPO) of polyunsaturated fatty acids in sperm cell membranes, induced by the production of reactive oxygen species during cryopreservation. It has been confirmed that frozen-thawed boar spermatozoa are susceptible to $FeSO_4$/ascorbate-induced LPO, measured by the production of malondialdehyde (MDA), which is capable of triggering apoptotic-like changes that could result in the sublethal sperm cryodamage [24, 30, 32]. Furthermore, the extent of LPO-induced damage to frozen-thawed spermatozoa can be analyzed by monitoring the colorimetric measurements of lipid peroxide formation with a fluorescent membrane probe, BODIPY$^{581/591}$-C11 [26, 30].

The sperm mitochondrial membrane potential is necessary for ATP production, which is the main energy support for several functions [25, 32]. Several studies showed that cryo-induced damage to the MMI of spermatozoa is one the major causes of their reduced fertilizing capacity [4, 5, 10, 24, 25, 29, 33]. These studies detected a marked deterioration in the sperm mitochondrial function following cryopreservation, as reported by the fluorescent staining with rhodamine 123 (R123), the lipophilic cationic compound 5,5′,6,6′-tetrachloro-1,1′,3,3′ tetraethylbenzymidazolyl carbocyanine iodine (JC-1), or with ATP measurements by the bioluminescence assay. The percentages of frozen-thawed spermatozoa with functional mitochondria, as assessed by either the R123/PI or JC-1/PI assay, are highly correlated to motility [5, 29, 33]. Besides the R123/PI and JC-1/PI assays, there are a plethora of fluorescent dyes that can be used to microscopically or cytometrically assess the sperm mitochondrial membrane function (MMF). Some fluorescent MitoTracker probes, such as MitoTracker Deep Red, MitoTracker Red, MitoTracker Orange, and MitoTracker Green, have been used effectively to assess the MMF on frozen-thawed spermatozoa [23, 26]. Boars with good and poor semen freezability ejaculates were identified using several sperm function parameters, including total and progressive motility (TMOT and PMOT, respectively), and rapid movement (RAP) analyzed by the computer-assisted semen analysis system, mitochondrial membrane function, MMF (JC-1/PI assay) and PMI (SYBR-14/PI assay) (**Figure 1**). Post-thaw analysis of the sperm parameters showed that boars with good semen freezability were characterized by significantly higher sperm cryosurvival (Boars 1–6) compared with those with poor semen freezability (Boars 7–10; **Figure 1**), suggesting the importance of these sperm parameters in the assessment of post-thaw semen quality (unpublished results).

2.3. Chromatin and DNA integrity

Sperm chromatin and DNA integrity is an uncompensable trait because abnormalities in the male genome, characterized by damaged chromatin/DNA structure, may be manifested until the sperm-oocyte fusion, or at early embryo development [34]. Accumulating evidence has shown that sperm DNA integrity is one of the parameters of semen quality assessment that has paramount importance in the prognosis of fertility and the outcome of assisted reproductive procedures [5, 34, 35,]. Among the most frequently used sperm DNA integrity assays are the Comet assay (SCGE), which quantifies double-stranded DNA (dsDNA) and single-stranded DNA (ssDNA) breaks under neutral or alkaline electrophoresis [8, 32, 35], the sperm chromatin structure assay (SCSA) measures the susceptibility of sperm chromatin to acid-induced denaturation in situ [34], and the terminal deoxynucleotidyl transferase-mediated dUDP nick end-labeling assay (TUNEL), which quantifies the incorporation of deoxyuridine triphosphate (dUTP) at ssDNA and dsDNA breaks [24, 34]. These DNA integrity assays have confirmed that the cryopreservation process increases the sperm susceptibility to DNA damage, irrespective of the extender or the protocol type [4, 5, 8, 21, 24, 32, 34, 35]. It is worth

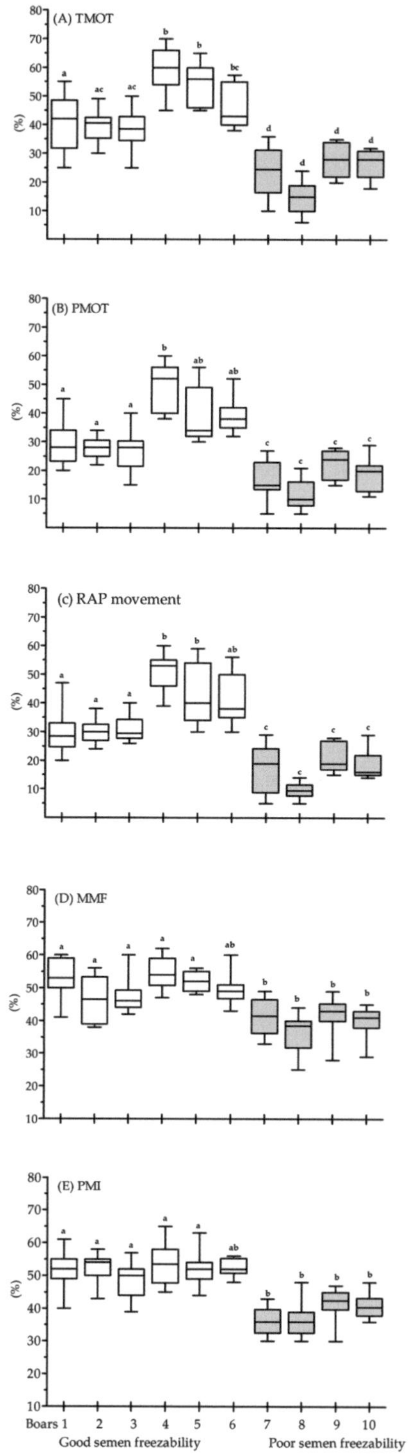

Figure 1. Distribution of the characteristics of frozen-thawed boar spermatozoa for: (A) Total sperm motility (TMOT). (B) Progressive sperm motility (PMOT). (C) Rapid moving (RAP) spermatozoa. (D) Mitochondrial membrane function (MMF). (E) Plasma membrane integrity (PMI) (*unpublished results*). The horizontal lines (–) indicate the medians with 25th and 75th percentile (boxes) and minimum-maximum values (*I*). Values with different letters (a–d) indicate a significant difference ($P < 0.05$).

noting that sperm DNA fragmentation is associated with differential expression of proteins in the viable sperm populations [36]. Intasqui et al. [36] postulated that the overexpression of the sperm proteins in the viable sperm population from ejaculates with high-sperm DNA fragmentation might indicate proteome alterations to compensate defects in sperm motility.

2.4. Protein freezability markers

Recently, seminal plasma and sperm proteins became an integral part of the reproductive area development. It is worth noting that proteins that are involved in the energy metabolism of spermatozoa play key roles in glycolysis, the citric acid cycle, and oxidative phosphorylation, which are required to provide sufficient energy for the sperm physiological functions [37]. The protein constellation of the SP and sperm cells, and their distinct subcompartments have been well documented in a numerous animal species, using a plethora of proteomic-based techniques [6, 37, 38]. While some specific sperm protein markers facilitating good semen freezability have been identified [10, 24, 39, 40], their function depends on the presence of mRNA that can be translated into proteins in the spermatozoa. Moreover, the differential expression patterns of certain classes of SP and sperm proteins following cryopreservation have been used as markers for semen freezability [3, 6, 10, 39–44]. Regarding boar semen, the physiological functions of SP and sperm proteins and their associations with freezability have been summarized in recent reviews by Yeste [3, 10]. In the bull, higher concentrations of a 26-kDa SP protein, known as lipocalin-type prostaglandin D synthase (L-PGDS), and a 13-kDa acidic seminal fluid protein (aSFP) were associated with high-fertility bulls, suggesting the importance of these proteins as freezability markers [41]. Moreover, a fertility-associated protein, osteopontin (OPN), an acidic glycoprotein occurring in the bovine SP, has been shown to induce capacitation and improve viability of spermatozoa by inhibiting the apoptotic pathways [39, 41]. Bovine SP proteins, collectively known as binder of sperm (BSP) proteins (BSP1, BSP 3, and BSP 5), bind to choline phospholipids in the sperm plasma membrane and are implicated in semen freezability [22, 39, 41, 42]. Recently, it has been confirmed that BSP1, one of the most abundantly expressed BSP proteins (representing approximately 25–47% of the total proteins in bovine SP), consists of four molecular forms that have varying cryoprotective effects on the bull spermatozoa [42]. According to Sarsaifi et al. [22], approximately 52% of the SP protein spots detected after cryopreservation were represented by four major protein fractions with different molecular weights, and 10 proteins, identified by mass spectrometry, were major bovine SP proteins. It is worth noting that two of these proteins, defined as phosphoglycerate kinase (PGK, 37–45 kDa) and phospholipase A2 (PLA2, 50–55 kDa), are implicated in glycolysis and the fertilization-associated processes, respectively [22]. More recently, it has been reported that the presence of fertility-associated 28–30-kDa heparin-binding proteins (HPBs) in bovine SP exerted better cryoprotective effects on the sperm structural and functional membrane integrity, which resulted in 13% higher conception rate than the bulls lacking the proteins in their SP [24]. Ledesma et al. [23] postulated that the decrease in phosphotyrosine signal of 45-, 40-, or 30-kDa protein in the presence of SP was concurrent with an inhibition of cryo-induced capacitation of ram spermatozoa, suggesting the relevance of these proteins as markers for the capacitation status of frozen-thawed spermatozoa.

Spermatozoa have a repertoire of distinct proteins localized in different subcellular structures that are associated with post-thaw semen quality [3, 6, 10, 40, 43]. In boar sperm extracts, the levels of outer dense fiber 2 (ODF2), A-kinase-anchoring protein 3 or 4 (AKAP3; AKAP4), heat-shock protein 90 (HSP90AA1), voltage-dependent anion channel 2 (VDAC2), acrosin-binding protein (ACRBP), and triosephosphate isomerase 1 (TP1) activities were associated with semen freezability [10, 40]. Furthermore, ODFs provide a stable and elastic structure to the flagellum of the spermatozoon, supporting its movement and protecting it during the epididymal transit and ejaculation [36, 39, 40]. The ODF2 seems to be essential to ODF assembly, and its overexpression in frozen-thawed boar spermatozoa was associated with reduced post-thaw semen quality [40]. Moreover, AKAP4 and AKAP3 occur in the fibrous sheath of sperm flagellum and are involved in sperm motility and morphology [36]. It has been confirmed that an increase in the expression of either AKAP4 or AKAP3 in frozen-thawed spermatozoa might be associated with their premature capacitation [40]. In another study, it has been demonstrated that greater levels of HSP90AA1 and VDAC2 in high-freezability boars might confer increased sperm cryotolerance [10]. Furthermore, greater expression levels of a fertility-associated protein, 90-kDa HSP (HSP90), were detected in bull spermatozoa with high cryotolerance and motility, indicating that the protein can be used as a marker for semen freezability [44]. The concept that HSPs supplementation to the freezing extender could protect spermatozoa against cryo-induced damage is supported by a report indicating that the HSPA8, a highly conserved member of the HSP70 family, exerted beneficial effects on post-thaw bull semen quality, as reflected by the reduced proportions of spermatozoa with apoptotic-like changes [45]. According to Chen et al. [40], higher levels of mRNA expression of the membrane proteins cytosolic SOD (Cu/Zn SOD1) in frozen-thawed boar semen might be due to the protective response of the sperm cells to cold stimulation and oxidation stress to prevent cryo-induced damage and also probably due to the toxicity of the components of the cryoprotectants. Recently, the application of high-throughput proteomics to the study of cryopreserved human semen showed substantial changes in the sperm proteome at every stage of the freezing-thawing processes [43]. Irrespective of the thawing procedure of frozen semen, it was reported that there was an increase in the expression levels of a few proteins, such as clusterin (CLU), histone H4 (HIST1H4A), and L-xylulose reductase (DCXR), whereas there was a decrease in the expression levels of several proteins, including apoptosis-inducing factor 1-mitochondrial (AIFM1), carbonic anhydrase 2 (CA2), acrosin (ACR), phosphoglycerate mutase 2 (PGAM2), inositol monophosphatase 1 (IMPA1), calmodulin (CALM1), cytochrome (CYC2), and NADH-cytochrome b5 reductase2 (CYB5R2) [43]. Besides the effect upon the sperm membrane protein P25b, an acrosome membrane-coating protein, cryopreservation causes a significant loss of several sperm-coating proteins, resulting in reduced post-thaw semen quality [10, 22–24, 39–45]. It appears that the cryo-induced decrease in the levels of sperm proteins is probably attributed to protein degradation, membrane damage due to osmotic stress, and the subsequent freezing-thawing causing the efflux of intracellular sperm constituents [6, 43]. Presently, the mechanism responsible for the cryo-induced increase in levels of protein expression is not fully understood, even though it has been suggested that enhanced phosphorylation might be a possible cause for abundance in some of the proteins following cryopreservation [23, 43]. Even though changes in the SP or sperm proteome could predict the cryotolerance of spermatozoa, they do not provide relevant information about possible associations of sperm transcript profiling with semen freezability.

3. Transcriptome studies on sperm-derived RNAs

The records of transcription of the late stages of sperm differentiation are easily accessible through sperm transcript fragments, which have the potential to be used as markers for fertility [13]. Among others, increasing focus has been given to the examination of the biological functions of mRNAs in spermatozoa of different animal species. It has been suggested that the analysis of the sperm-derived RNAs might provide potential links between the sperm proteome and semen freezability [17, 18, 20, 46–48]. It should be underlined that the isolation of high-quality RNAs from fresh or frozen-thawed semen is important to assess the sperm gene expression [19, 46, 49, 50]. However, to optimize the isolation protocol of total RNA from spermatozoa of different animal species, the procedure has to be modified, and should incorporate a quality control reverse transcription polymerase chain reaction (RT-PCR) to avoid somatic cell contamination [17, 19, 46, 49]. Presently, human sperm transcripts are the best characterized among all mammals with respect to RNA sequence profiling. Even though microarray techniques, coupled with either quantitative real-time qPCR or qRT-PCR, have revealed limited features of the transcriptome and global patterns of gene expression in spermatozoa, these techniques have revealed that sperm transcripts affecting different metabolic pathways are related to semen fertility [48, 49, 51–54]. A study based on the evaluation of sperm capacitation status provides evidence, indicating that the sperm-derived RNAs can be translated *de novo* using mitochondrial-type ribosomes, and at least 26 such sperm-translated proteins are known to be required during capacitation, sperm-egg interactions, and fertilization [11, 54].

Recently, the utilization of advanced molecular genetics tools has led to a rapid development of high-throughput RNA-Seq techniques, which have been used to explore the relationship between sperm functions with the transcript profiles of raw fresh or frozen-thawed spermatozoa [12, 50]. The resolution of RNA population has been optimized with the utilization of next-generation sequencing (NGS) technology, to uncover complete transcript profiles of mammalian spermatozoa [12], making significant contributions to elucidate the physiological roles of sperm-derived RNAs. Moreover, the wider adaption of RNA-Seq has revealed a complex RNA repertoire in spermatozoa from different animal species, including the bull [17, 51–53, 55, 56], boar [46–48], and stallion [54]. However, despite the increasingly wide applications of RNA-Seq in the analysis of different cellular tissues, its application is limited to screening of the mRNA profiles of frozen-thawed spermatozoa to uncover candidate genes associated with semen freezability.

Despite its apparent transcriptionally inert state, a mature spermatozoon contains diverse populations of both small and large RNAs [11–13, 47, 55]. Since their discovery in 1989, sperm-derived RNAs were implicated in spermatogenesis and in fertilization and early embryonic development, suggesting that they are not merely the remnants of sperm cell development [11, 46, 54]. Notwithstanding the rich repertoire of coding and noncoding RNAs in mammalian spermatozoa, they are not a random remnant from spermatogenesis in testes, but a selectively retained and functionally coherent collection of RNAs [12, 54, 55]. Spermatozoa contain complex populations of RNAs, including several stable full-length RNAs and a variety of different RNAs, such as ribosome RNAs (rRNA), mitochondrial RNAs (mtRNAs), miRNAs (18–24 nucleotides), piwi-interacting RNAs (piRNAs, 26–31 nucleotides), and small interfering RNAs (siRNAs), which originate from double-stranded RNAs (dsRNAs) [11–17, 55]. The precise population of mRNAs in spermatozoa is unknown, but has been estimated to be about 3000–7000 transcripts [17, 54]. It has been established that a majority of sperm mRNAs are located in the nucleus, and a limited number of mRNAs are located in other areas, such as the mid-piece region and flagella fibrous sheath [11]. Individual identified sperm transcripts include mRNAs for ribosomal and mitochondrial proteins, protamines, and proteins involved in signal transduction and cell proliferation [13].

Screening of differentially expressed genes (DEGs) in spermatozoa has been explored mainly to investigate the associations of the gene expression levels with male fertility [11, 14]. Using microarray-based techniques, significant differences in the expression of two genes—testis-specific protein1 (*TPX-1*) and lactate dehydrogenase C, transcript variant (*LDHC*)—were detected in human spermatozoa with high and low motilities [11]. Accumulating evidence has been shown that the coding and noncoding RNAs in spermatozoa play an important role in chromatin stabilization, facilitating the selective escape of sequences necessary for early development from re-packaging by protamines [12, 52, 55]. In human spermatozoa, some putatively sperm transcripts associated with male fertility and early embryo development include *CLU*, *AKAP4*, Protamine 1 (*PRM1*), Protamine 2 (*PRM2*), and heat-shock-binding protein1 (*HSBP1*) [11]. It has been reported that *CLU* binds to the plasma membrane and is the main protein that has been overexpressed in individuals from the low-sperm DNA fragmentation group [36]. Even though the potential role of *CLU* in sperm function is still obscure, it has the potential to be a fertility biomarker for bull, stallion, or human semen [36]. Besides the crucial roles of DEGs in sperm function, there is limited information about the effects of the cryopreservation process on their expression levels. Several full-length transcripts have been identified in the frozen-thawed bull spermatozoa using RNA-Seq [17, 55]. In frozen-thawed bull spermatozoa, highly abundant full-length transcripts, such as *PRM1*, phospholipase C zeta 1 (*PLCZ*1), cysteine-rich secretory protein 2 (*CRISP2*), and calmegin 1 (*CLGN1*), which have been involved in capacitation and fertilization, had been identified using the RNA-Seq [17]. A previous study showed that the transcripts encoding for a serine/threonine testis-specific protein kinase (*TSSK6*) and a metalloproteinase non-coding RNA (*ADAM5P*) were associated with high-motility status in the bull [51].

Significant differences were detected in the DEGs between fresh and frozen-thawed bull spermatozoa using microarray technique in conjunction with qRT-PCR analysis and that upregulations of several DEGs existed, such as ribosomal protein L31 (*RPL31*) and glutamate-cysteine ligase catalytic subunit (*GCLC*), probably due to the protective response of spermatozoa to cold shock and oxidation stress conditions [56]. More recently, an abundance of DEGs has been shown to be highly expressed in bull spermatozoa with poor post-thaw motility compared with those with good post-thaw motility [53]. According to Yathish et al. [53], some of the significantly upregulated DEGs in poor motility freezability ejaculates included the cytochrome b5 reductase 4 (C*YB5R4*), which regulates stress-induced ROS production in spermatozoa; the chaperonin containing T-complex polypeptide 1, subunit 5 (*CCT5*) that is involved in proper folding of cytoskeletal proteins and its high expression is associated with spermatogenesis dysfunction; and *PACSIN3* (protein kinase C and casein kinase substrate in neurons), which is involved in the maintenance of the physiological function of membrane proteins. In a recent study, the RNA-Seq has detected differences in mRNA transcripts of frozen-thawed semen between high-fertility and low-fertility bulls, and several of these transcripts were considered unique to either fertility group, which differed in their biological functions, such as enrichment of regulatory transcripts for growth and protein kinase activity in the high-fertility bulls [55]. Card et al. [55] demonstrated that the sperm transcript cytochrome oxidase subunit 7C (*COX7C*), which is involved in the terminal step in the electron transport chain leading to ATP synthesis in the inner mitochondrial membrane, was negatively correlated with bull fertility. The authors hypothesized that the abundant expression of COX7C in frozen-thawed spermatozoa from the low-fertility bulls might represent inefficient translation of the transcript, resulting in impaired mitochondrial function during the later stages of spermatogenesis. Similarly, inefficient translation of protein synthesis has been suggested as a possible cause for other sperm transcripts that were abundantly expressed in the low-fertility bulls [55]. However, it should be emphasized that both *PRM1* and *PRM2* are among the most strongly associated transcripts with different semen quality parameters, such as sperm concentration, motility, morphology, and chromatin and DNA integrity, as well as with fertility and embryo quality [11, 17, 46, 52, 55]. Significant reduction in the expression levels of *PRM1* mRNA transcript in post-thaw bull semen was concurrent with compromised progressive sperm motility [52]. It appears that dysfunction in protein synthesis might be associated with aberrant mRNA retention, indicating that the regulation of protamine translation might compromise fertility [11, 52]. Further study, coupling qRT-PCR analysis with an enzyme-linked immunosorbent assay (ELISA), showed that the cryopreservation process caused significant changes in the expression levels of several sperm-derived mRNAs and proteins of epigenetic-related genes in boar spermatozoa [48]. Evidence has been shown that the mRNA expression levels of *PRM1* and *PRM2* were significantly decreased in frozen-thawed bull spermatozoa [52], thus reinforcing the findings of different studies, and indicating that the cryopreservation process induces sperm DNA damage [4, 5, 21, 24, 32, 34, 35]. According to Zeng et al. [48], the mRNA expression levels of *Dnmt3a* and *Dnmt3b*, which are DNA methyl transferases known to possess *de novo* methylation activity in mammalian cells, were markedly suppressed in frozen-thawed spermatozoa, reaffirming the unfavorable effects of the cryopreservation process on post-thaw sperm survival. Furthermore, different transcripts of HSPs have been detected in spermatozoa of various animal species, particularly the most abundantly expressed 70-kDa HSP, which is an effective marker for sperm cryotolerance and might be associated with post-thaw semen quality [45, 57]. Furthermore, seasonality is an important factor that affects the mRNA profiles of boar spermatozoa, resulting in marked differences in the expression levels of genes, which are implicated in numerous sperm physiological and biochemical functions [47]. These findings corroborate those of a recent study, indicating that the marked differences in the gene expression profiles of SP and sperm proteome, in response to seasonal changes, significantly affected the biochemical composition of boar semen, which could compromise post-thaw semen quality [58].

Currently, the biological roles of small-nuclear RNAs (snRNAs)—miRNAs, piRNAs, and siRNAs—which are expressed specifically and abundantly in spermatogenic cells, have been documented by several authors [11–17]. Quantitative RT-PCR analysis on boar sperm RNA revealed that the mRNA targets of the differentially expressed miRNAs encode proteins previously described to play specific roles in sperm function, such as motility and capacitation [14]. According to Chang et al. [16], the differential expression of 15 miRNAs between the cauda epididymal spermatozoa and fresh ejaculate in the boar suggests that significant mRNA expression and miRNA regulation are implicated in apoptosis, and are associated with the sperm maturation processes. The authors postulated that the targeted gene, adrenoceptor beta 2 (*ADRB2*), a member of the G-protein-coupled receptor superfamily, activates adenylyl cyclase leading to the activation of cAMP-dependent kinase, whereas another targeted gene, the adenylate cyclase 3 (*ADCY3*), catalyzes the formation of the second messenger cAMP, which in turn leads to elevated cAMP levels. It should be emphasized that while many miRNAs are conserved among different animal species, some of them are species-specific [12]. Furthermore, profiling of the SP by Illumina high-throughput sequencing showed that piRNA appears to play more important and direct roles in spermatogenesis and male infertility, and its expression was significantly reduced in the SP of infertile patients compared with the healthy individuals [12, 13, 15]. However, it remains unclear how individual miRNAs and siRNAs in spermatozoa function at the molecular levels, and the impact of the cryopreservation process on their biological functions. It should be emphasized that the SP and mature spermatozoa contain a plethora of other small RNAs in which their roles in sperm function are currently unknown [13].

4. Concluding remarks

Even though proteins of the SP and spermatozoa have been used as semen freezability markers, these expectations are over-shadowed by the problems associated with the inherent male variability in sperm cryosurvival. The search for a new set of freezability markers using transcriptome studies on RNA-Seq data, bioinformatics study, and proteome characterization of protein expression patterns in frozen-thawed spermatozoa will offer new perspectives to enhance the marker-assisted selection programs in animal breeding. It is envisaged that such freezability markers will also help to unravel the biological functions of sperm-derived mRNA transcripts in the mechanism underlying cryotolerance of spermatozoa from various domestic animal species, and will have a significant impact in the technology of semen cryopreservation.

Acknowledgements

This study was supported by a research project from the National Science Centre, Poland (2015/19/B/NZ9/01333).

Author details

Leyland Fraser

Address all correspondence to: fraser@uwm.edu.pl

Department of Animal Biochemistry and Biotechnology, Faculty of Animal Bioengineering, University of Warmia and Mazury in Olsztyn, Olsztyn, Poland

References

[1] Benson JD, Woods EJ, Walters EM, Crister JK. The cryobiology of spermatozoa. Theriogenology. 2012;**78**(8):1682-1699. DOI: 10.1016/j.theriogenology.2012.06.007

[2] Prien S, Iacovides S. Cryoprotectants & cryopreservation of equine semen: A review of industry cryoprotectants and the effects of cryopreservation on equine semen membranes. Journal of Dairy, Veterinary & Animal Research. 2016;**3**(1):00063, 1-8. DOI: 10.15406/jdvar.2016.03.00063

[3] Yeste M. Recent advances in boar sperm cryopreservation: State of the art and current perspectives. Reproduction in Domestic Animals. 2015;**50**(Suppl 2):71-79. DOI: 10.1111/rda.12569

[4] Castro LS, Hamilton TR, Mendes CM, Nichi M, Barnabe VH, Visintin JA, Assumpção ME. Sperm cryodamage occurs after rapid freezing phase: Flow cytometry approach and antioxidant enzymes activity at different stages of cryopreservation. Journal of Animal Science and Biotechnology. 2016;**5**(7):1-9. DOI: 10.1186/s40104-016-0076-x

[5] Gürler H, Malama E, Heppelmann M, Calisici O, Leiding C, Kastelic JP, Bollwein H. Effects of cryopreservation on sperm viability, synthesis of reactive oxygen species and DNA damage of bovine sperm. Theriogenology. 2016;**86**:562-571. DOI: 10.1016/j.theriogenology.2016.02.007

[6] Leahy T, Gadella BM. Sperm surface changes and physiological consequences induced by sperm handling and storage. Reproduction. 2011;**142**:759-778. DOI: 10.1530/REP-11-0310

[7] Thurston LM, Siggins K, Mileham AJ, Watson PF, Holt WV. Identification of amplified restriction fragment length polymorphism markers linked to genes controlling boar sperm viability following cryopreservation. Biology of Reproduction. 2002;**66**(3):545-554. DOI: 10.1095/biolreprod66.3.545

[8] Fraser L, Pareek CS, Strzeżek J. Identification of amplified fragment length polymorphism (AFLP) markers associated with freezability of boar semen – a preliminary study. Medycyna Weterynaryjna. 2008;**64**:646-649

[9] Roca J, Broekhuijse MLWJ, Parrilla I, Rodríguez-Martínez H, EA Martinez EA, Bolarin A. Boar differences in artificial insemination outcomes: Can they be minimized? Reproduction in Domestic Animals. 2015;**50**(Suppl. 2):48-55. DOI: 10.1111/rda.12530

[10] Yeste M. Sperm cryopreservation update: Cryodamage, markers, and factors affecting the sperm freezability in pigs. Theriogenology. 2016;**85**:47-64. DOI: 10.1016/j.theriogenology.2015.09.047

[11] Dadoune JP. Spermatozoal RNAs. What about their functions? Microscopy Research and Technique. 2009;**72**:536-551. DOI: 10.1002/jemt.20697

[12] Jodar M, Selvaraju S, Sendler E, Diamond MP, Krawetz SA. The presence, role and clinical use of spermatozoal RNAs. Human Reproduction Update. 2013;**19**:604-624. DOI: 10.1093/humupd/dmt031.

[13] Casas E, Vavouri T. Sperm epigenomics: Challenges and opportunities. Frontiers in Genetics. 2014;5:Article 330, 1-7. DOI: 10.3389/fgene.2014.00330

[14] Curry E, Safranski TJ, Pratta SL. Differential expression of porcine sperm microRNAs and their association with sperm morphology and motility. Theriogenology. 2011;**76**:1532-1539. DOI: 10.1016/j.theriogenology.2011.06.025

[15] Hong Y, Wang C, Fu Z, Liang H, Zhang S, Lu M, Sun W, Ye C, Zhang CY, Zen K, Shi L, Zhang C, Chen X. Systematic characterization of seminal plasma piRNAs as molecular biomarkers for male infertility. Scientific Reports. 2016;**6**:24229, 1-10. DOI: 10.1038/srep24229

[16] Chang Y, Dai DH, Li Y, Zhang Y, Zhang M, Zhou GB, Zeng CJ. Differences in the expression of microRNAs and their predicted gene targets between cauda epididymal and ejaculated boar sperm. Theriogenology. 2016;**86**(9):2162-2171. DOI: 10.1016/j.theriogenology.2016.07.012

[17] Card CJ, Anderson EJ, Zamberlan S, Krieger KE, Kaproth M, Sartini BL. Cryopreserved bovine spermatozoal transcript profile as revealed by high-throughput ribonucleic acid sequencing. Biology of Reproduction. 2013;**88**(1):1-9. DOI: 10.1095/biolreprod.112.103788

[18] Fraser L. A novel approach to assess semen freezability. Veterinary Medicine – Open Journal. 2016;**1**(2):e5-e6. DOI: 10.17140/VMOJ-1-e003

[19] Fraser L, Brym P, Pareek CS. Isolation of total RNA from fresh and frozen-thawed boar semen and its relevance in transcriptome studies. South African Journal of Animal Science. 2017;**47**(1):56-60. DOI: 10.4314/sajas.v47i1.5

[20] Fraser L. Sperm transcriptome profiling for assessment of boar semen freezability. IJASRM. 2016;**1**(12):9-12

[21] Kumar D, Kumar P, Singh P, Yadav SP, Sarkar SK, Bharadwaj A, Yadav PS. Characteristics of frozen thawed semen in predicting the fertility of buffalo bulls. Indian Journal of Animal Science. 2014;**84**(4):389-392

[22] Sarsaifi K, Vejayan J, Haron AW, Yusoff R, Hani H, Rasoli M, Omar MA, Othman AM. Protein profile and functionality of spermatozoa from two semen collection methods in Bali bulls. Life Science. 2015;**172**:96-105. DOI: 10.1016/j.livsci.2014.12.004

[23] Ledesma A, Fernández-Alegre E, Cano A, Hozbor F, Martínez-Pastor F, Cesarid A. Seminal plasma proteins interacting with sperm surface revert capacitation indicators in frozen-thawed ram sperm. Animal Reproduction Science. 2016;**173**:35-41. DOI: 10.1016/j.anireprosci.2016.08.007

[24] Karunakaran M, Devanathan TG. Evaluation of bull semen for fertility-associated protein, in vitro characters and fertility. Journal of Applied Animal Research. 2017;**45**(1):136-144. DOI: 10.1080/09712119.2015.1129343

[25] Wasilewska K, Zasiadczyk Ł, Fraser L, Mogielnicka-Brzozowska M, Kordan W. The benefits of cooling boar semen in different long-term extenders prior to cryopreservation on sperm quality characteristics. Reproduction in Domestic Animals. 2016;**51**(5):781-788. DOI: 10.1111/rda.12751

[26] Hossain MdS, Johannisson A, Wallgren M, Nagy S, Siqueira AP, Rodríguez-Martinez H. Flow cytometry for the assessment of animal sperm integrity and functionality: State of the art. Asian Journal of Andrology. 2011;**13**:406-419. DOI: 10.1038/aja.2011.15

[27] Nagy S, Jansen J, Topper EK, Gadella BM. A triple-stain flow cytometric method to assess plasma- and acrosome-membrane integrity of cryopreserved bovine sperm immediately after thawing in presence of egg-yolk particles. Biology of Reproduction. 2003;**68**:1828-1835. DOI: 10.1095/biolreprod.102.011445

[28] Peña FJ. Detecting subtle changes in sperm membranes in veterinary andrology. Asian Journal of Andrology. 2007;**9**:731-737. DOI: 10.1111/j.1745-7262.2007.00311.x

[29] Yoon SJ, Kwon WS, Rahman MdS, Lee JS, Pang GM. A novel approach to identifying physical markers of cryo-damage in bull spermatozoa. PLoS One. 2015;**10**(5):e0126232. DOI: 10.1371/journal.pone.0126232

[30] Ferrusola O, Fernández LG, Morrell JM, Sandoval CS, Garcia BM, Tapia JA, Rodríguez-Martínez H, Tapia JA, Peña FJ. Lipid peroxidation, assessed with BODIPY-C_{11}, increases after cryopreservation of stallion spermatozoa, is stallion-dependent and is related to apoptotic-like changes. Reproduction. 2009;**138**:55-63. DOI: 10.1530/REP-08-0484

[31] Pinart E, Yeste M, Bonet S. Acrosin activity is a good predictor of boar sperm freezability. Theriogenology. 2015;**83**:1525-533. DOI: 10.1016/j.theriogenology.2015.02.005

[32] Fraser L, Zasiadczyk Ł, Pareek CS. Effects of boar variability on comet-detected sperm DNA damage following cryopreservation. Animal Production Science. 2016. DOI: 10.1071/AN16274

[33] Fraser L, Dziekońska A, Strzeżek R, Strzeżek J. Dialysis of boar semen prior to freezing thawing: Its effects on post-thaw sperm characteristics. Theriogenology. 2007;**67**:994-1003. DOI: 10.1016/j.theriogenology.2006.12.002

[34] Evenson DP. The sperm chromatin structure assay (SCSA®) and other sperm DNA fragmentation tests for evaluation of sperm nuclear DNA integrity as related to fertility. Animal Reproduction Science. 2016;**169**:56-75. DOI: 10.1016/j.anireprosci.2016.01.017

[35] Fraser L, Parda A, Filipowicz K, Strzeżek J. Comparison of post-thaw DNA integrity of boar spermatozoa assessed with the neutral Comet assay and sperm-Sus Halomax test kit. Reproduction in Domestic Animals. 2010;**45**:e155-e160. DOI: 10.1111/j.1439-0531.2009.01537.x

[36] Intasqui P, Camargo M, Del Giudice PT, Spaine DM, Carvalho VM, Cardozo KHM, Cedenho AP, Bertolla RP. Unraveling the sperm proteome and post-genomic pathways associated with sperm nuclear DNA fragmentation. Journal of Assisted Reproduction and Genetics. 2013;**30**:1187-1120. DOI: 10.1007/s10815-013-0054-6

[37] Holland A, Ohlendieck K. Comparative profiling of the sperm proteome. Proteomics. 2015;**15**:632-648. DOI: 10.1002/pmic.201400032

[38] Perez-Patiño C, Barranco I, Parrilla I, Valero ML, Martinez EA, Rodriguez-Martinez H, Roca J. Characterization of the porcine seminal plasma proteome comparing ejaculate portions. Journal of Proteomics. 2016;**142**:15-23. DOI: 10.1016/j.jprot.2016.04.026

[39] Moura AA, Memili E. Functional aspects of seminal plasma and sperm proteins and their potential as molecular markers of fertility. Animal Reproduction. 2016;**13**(3):191-199. DOI:10.21451/19843143-AR884

[40] Chen X, Zhu H, Hu C, Hao H, Zhang J, Li K, Zhao X, Qin T, Zhao K, Zhu H, Wang D. Identification of differentially expressed proteins in fresh and frozen–thawed boar spermatozoa by iTRAQ-coupled 2D LC–MS/MS. Reproduction. 2014;**147**:321-330. DOI: 10.1530/REP-130313

[41] Kumar P, Kumar D, Singh I, Yadav PS. Seminal plasma proteome: Promising biomarkers for bull fertility. Agricultural Research. 2012;**1**(1):78-86. DOI: 10.1007/s40003-011-0006-2

[42] Magalhães MJ Jr, Martins LF, Senra RL, Santos TF, Okano DS, Pereira PR, Faria-Campos A, Campos SV, Guimarães JD, Baracat-Pereira MC. Differential abundances of four forms of Binder of SPerm 1 in the seminal plasma of *Bos taurus in*dicus bulls with different patterns of semen freezability. Theriogenology. 2016;**86**(3):766-777. DOI: 10.1016/j.theriogenology.2016.02.030

[43] Bogle OA, Kumar K, Attardo-Parrinello C, Lewis SEM, Estanyol JM, Ballesc JL, Oliva R. Identification of protein changes in human spermatozoa throughout the cryopreservation process. Andrology. 2017;**5**:10-22. DOI: 10.1111/andr.12279

[44] Wang P, Wang YF, Wang H, Wang CW, Zan LS, Hu JH, Li QW, Jia YH, Guo-Ji Ma GJ. HSP90 expression correlation with the freezing resistance of bull sperm. Zygote. 2014;**22**:239-245. DOI: 10.1017/S096719941300004x

[45] Holt WV, Del Valle DI, Fazeli A. Heat shock protein A8 stabilizes the bull sperm plasma membrane during cryopreservation: Effects of breed, protein concentration, and mode of use. Theriogenology. 2015;**84**:693-701. DOI: 10.1016/j.theriogenology.2015.05.004

[46] Yang CC, Lin YS, Hsu CC, Wu SC, Lin EC, Cheng WTK. Identification and sequencing of remnant messenger RNAs found in domestic swine (*Sus scrofa*) fresh ejaculated spermatozoa. Animal Reproduction Science. 2009;**113**:143-155. DOI: 10.1016/j.anireprosci.2008.08.012

[47] Yang CC, Lin YS, Hsu CC, Tsai MH, Wu SC, Cheng WTK. Seasonal effect on sperm messenger RNA profile of domestic swine (*Sus Scrofa*). Animal Reproduction Science. 2010;**119**(1-2):76-84. DOI: 10.1016/j.anireprosci.2009.12.002

[48] Zeng C, Peng W, Ding L, He L, Zhang Y, Fang D, Tang K. A preliminary study on epigenetic changes during boar spermatozoa cryopreservation. Cryobiology. 2014;**69**:119-127. DOI: 10.1016/j.cryobiol.2014.06.003

[49] Han CM, Chen R, Li T, Chen XL, Zheng YF, Ma MT, Gao QH. Evaluation of the semen swim-up method for bovine sperm RNA extraction. Genetics and Molecular Research. 2016;**15**(2):1-9. DOI: 10.4238/gmr.15027713

[50] Schuster A, Tang C, Xie Y, Ortogero N, Yuan S, Yan W. SpermBase – A database for sperm borne RNA contents. Biology of Reproduction. 2016;**95**(5):99, 1-12. DOI: 10.1095/biolreprod.116.142190

[51] Bissonnette N, Levesque-Sergerie JP, Thibault C, Boissonneault G. Spermatozoal transcriptome profiling for bull sperm motility: A potential tool to evaluate semen quality. Reproduction. 2009;**38**:65-80. DOI: 10.1530/REP-08-0503

[52] Ganguly I, Gaur GK, Kumar S, Mandal DK, Kumar M, Singh U, Kumar S, Sharma A. Differential expression of protamine 1 and 2 genes in mature spermatozoa of normal and motility impaired semen producing crossbred Frieswal (HF × Sahiwal) bulls. Research in Veterinary Science. 2013;**94**:256-262. DOI: 10.1016/j.rvsc.2012.09.001

[53] Yathish HM, Kumar S, Dubey PP, Modi RP, Chaudhary R, Kumar AS, Ghosh SK, Sarkar M, Sivamani B. Profiling of sperm gene transcripts in crossbred (*Bos taurus* × *Bos indicus*) bulls. Animal Reproduction Science. 2017;**177**:25-35. DOI: 10.1016/j.anireprosci.2016.12.003

[54] Das PJ, McCarthy F, Vishnoi M, Paria N, Gresham C, Gang L, Kachroo P, Sudderth AK, Teague S, Love CC, Varner DD, Chowdhary BP, Raudsepp T. Stallion sperm transcriptome comprises functionally coherent coding and regulatory RNAs as revealed by microarray analysis and RNA seq. PLoS One. 2013;**8**(2):1-15, e56535. DOI:10.1371/journal.pone.0056535

[55] Card CJ, Kreiger KE, Kaproth M, Sartini BL. Oligo-dT selected spermatozoal transcript profiles differ among higher and lower fertility dairy sires. Animal Reproduction Science. 2017;**177**:105-123. DOI: 10.1016/j.anireprosci.2016.12.011

[56] Chen X, Wang Y, Zhu H[1], Hao H, Zhao X, Qin T, Wang D. Comparative transcript profiling of gene expression of fresh and frozen-thawed bull sperm. Theriogenology. 2015;**4**:504-511. DOI: 10.1016/j.theriogenology.2014.10.015

[57] Zhang XG, Hong JY, Yan GJ, Wang YF, Li QW, Hu JH. Association of *heat shock protein 70* with motility of frozen-thawed sperm in bulls. Czech Journal of Animal Science. 2015;**60**(6):256-262. DOI: 10.17221/8239-CJAS

[58] Fraser L, Strzeżek J, Filipowicz K, Mogielnicka-Brzozowska M, Zasiadczyk Ł. Age and seasonal-dependent variations in the biochemical composition of boar semen. Theriogenology. 2016;**86**:806-816. DOI: 10.1016/j.theriogenology.2016.02.035

Chapter 4

Mitigation of the Heat Stress Impact in Livestock Reproduction

Govindan Krishnan, Madiajagan Bagath,
Prathap Pragna, Mallenahally Kusha Vidya,
Joy Aleena, Payyanakkal Ravindranathan Archana,
Veerasamy Sejian and Raghavendra Bhatta

Additional information is available at the end of the chapter

http://dx.doi.org/10.5772/intechopen.69091

Abstract

Heat stress affects the fertility and reproductive livestock performance by compromising the physiology reproductive tract, through hormonal imbalance, decreased oocyte quality and poor semen quality, and decreased embryo development and survival. Heat stress decreases the secretion of luteinizing hormone and estradiol resulting in reduced length and intensity of estrus expression, increased incidence of anoestrus and silent heat in farm animals. Oocytes exposed to thermal stress lose its competence for fertilization and development into the blastocyst stage, which results in decreased fertility because of the production of poor quality oocytes and embryos. Furthermore, low progesterone secretion limits the endometrial functions, and subsequently embryo development. In addition, the increased secretion of endometrial prostaglandin F2 alpha during heat stress threatens the maintenance of pregnancy. In general, the percentage of conception rate was found to be reduced by 4.6% for each unit increase in temperature humidity index (THI) above 70, and heat stress during pregnancy further slows down the growth of the foetus and results in lower birth weight. In tropical and subtropical regions, during hot days, the testicular temperature may increase and impair both the spermatogenic cycle and semen quality, which culminates in decreased bull fertility. The effects of heat stress on livestock can be minimized via adapting suitable scientific strategies comprising physical modifications of the environment, nutritional management and genetic development of breeds that are less sensitive to heat stress. In addition, the summer infertility may be countered through advanced reproductive technologies involving hormonal treatments, timed artificial insemination and embryo transfer, which may enhance the chances for establishing pregnancy in farm animals.

Keywords: antioxidants, cooling devices, estrus, fertility, shade, thermo-tolerant genes

1. Introduction

The performance, health, and well-being of livestock are strongly affected by climate. High ambient temperatures, high direct and indirect solar radiation and humidity are environmental stressing factors that impose a strain on animals. Among the environmental variables affecting livestock, heat stress seems to be one of the most intriguing factors hampering animal production in many regions of the world. Even though new knowledge on the animal responses to the environment continually arises, managing livestock to reduce the impact of climate remains a challenge. Considerable efforts are, therefore, needed from livestock researchers to counter the impact of environmental stresses on livestock production. Besides ensuring the livelihood security to our poor and marginal farmers, stress mitigation can also improve the economy of livestock industry as a whole. Hence, it is crucial to understand the impact of environmental stress on livestock production and reproduction. These efforts may help in identifying the appropriate targets for developing suitable mitigation strategies.

Thermal stress effects on livestock are of multifactorial nature. It directly alters and impairs the cellular functions in various tissues of the body and the redistribution of blood flow, as well as the reduction in food intake, which ultimately results in reduced production performance. Reproductive functions of livestock are particularly vulnerable to climate change; it has been established that large ruminants are more prone to heat stress compared with small ruminants [1]. Heat stress is the major cause for infertility and reproductive inefficiency in livestock, resulting in profound economic losses. Heat stress reduces the libido, fertility and embryonic survival in livestock and favors the occurrence of diseases in neonates with reduced immunity. Heat stress affects the fertility and reproductive performance of livestock species through compromising the functions of the reproductive tract, disrupting the hormonal balance, decreasing the oocyte quality, and thereby decreasing embryo development and survival [2–4]. In the tropical and subtropical regions, during the hot season, both the poor quality of oocytes and embryos results in decreased conception rate and subsequently with more days open resulting in huge economic losses to the dairy industry [5]. The high ambient temperature and relative humidity directly affect reproduction by altering or impairing various tissues or organs of the reproductive system of animal [6]. The threshold level of temperature humidity index (THI) for the high performance in terms of milk yield and reproduction is around THI 72 in tropical and subtropical climates. However, recent studies on THI in temperate climate emphasized that the THI lower than 68 is suitable for cattle performance and welfare [7].

This chapter is an attempt to cover in detail the impact of various heat stress factors on livestock reproduction, in both the female and male. Apart from these influences, the chapter also elaborates on available mitigation strategies directed to sustain livestock reproduction in the changing climate scenario.

2. Impact of heat stress on female reproduction

High environmental temperatures impair the female reproductive process at various stages of pubertal development, conception and embryonic mortality. Stress inhibits the reproductive performance of livestock species by activating the hypothalamic-pituitary-adrenal (HPA) axis, which subsequently excites the pituitary gland to release adrenocorticotropic hormone (ATCH) (**Figure 1**). The ACTH stimulates the release of glucocorticoids and catecholamines, which act extensively to alleviate the effect of stress. However, ACTH-stimulated glucocorticoid release is responsible for an inhibitory effect on the reproductive axis. Heat stress reduces the length and intensity of estrus, alters follicular development and increases the rate of apoptosis in the antral and pre-antral follicles. Extreme environmental temperatures delay the onset of puberty in male and female animals. Furthermore, heat stress during follicular recruitment suppresses the subsequent growth and development to ovulation [8]. Changes in the follicular growth disturb further progress and function of the oocytes [9, 10]. The chronic release of ACTH, such as the associated with heat stress, inhibits the ovulation and follicular development by altering the efficiency of follicular selection and dominance and glucocorticoids are critical to mediating this inhibitory effect on reproduction [11]. Further, high level of glucocorticoids during heat stress directly inhibits the meiotic maturation of oocytes, and, in addition, corticotropic releasing hormone (CRH) inhibits the ovarian steroidogenesis, derived of the decrease in the secretion of luteinizing hormone (LH). The consequent decrease in estradiol results in reduced length and intensity of estrus expression [12].

2.1. Reproductive hormones in female livestock

The reproductive hormones play a vital role as they regulate various stages of development and function in the female reproductive system. The high ambient temperature and solar

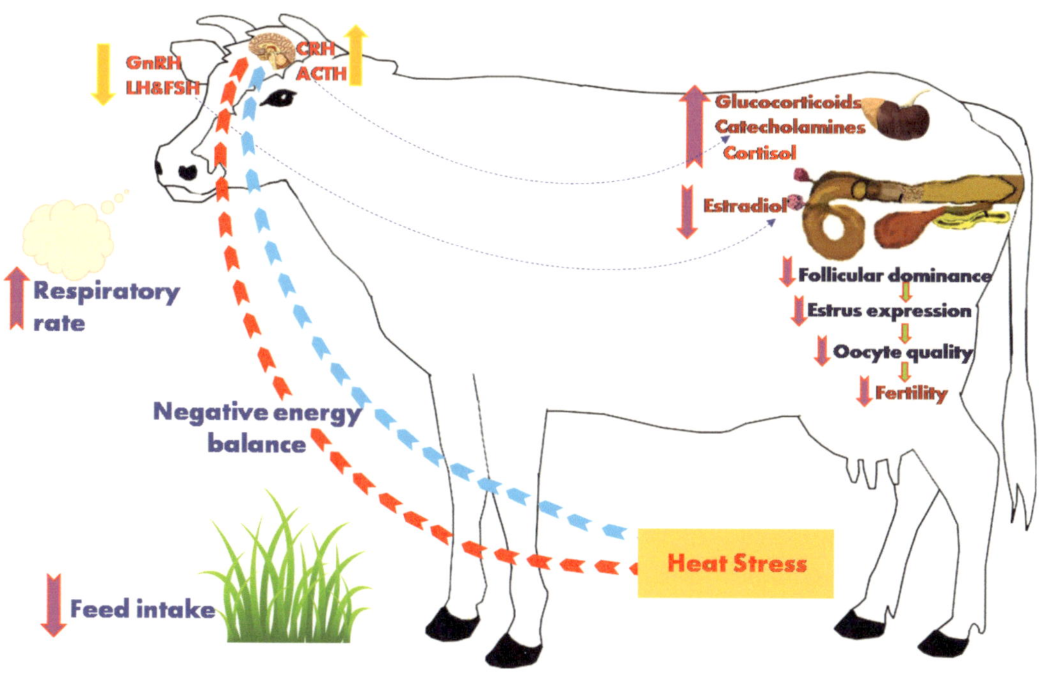

Figure 1. Impact of heat stress on female reproductive performance.

radiation as a result of climate change may affect the reproductive rhythm via the hypothalamic-hypophyseal-ovarian axis [13]. Various studies also revealed a significant negative correlation between environmental temperature and the reproductive hormone concentration, which in turn cause compromised reproductive efficiency in farm animals [14, 15]. The foremost important factors that regulate the ovarian activity are the gonadotropin-releasing hormone (GnRH), from the hypothalamus, and the gonadotropins (FSH and LH), from anterior hypophysis.

In cattle, the immediate 16 h exposure to a higher temperature (40°C) on day 12 of the estrous cycle lead to a significant reduction of GnRH-induced FSH secretion [16], whereas tonic FSH secretion was elevated probably due to reduced inhibition of negative feedback from small follicles [8]. Heat stress decreases LH pulse amplitude and frequency in cattle with low estradiol, thereby compromising the maturation and ovulation of the dominant follicles, while low tonic LH levels also hinder luteal development by inhibiting follicular growth and turnover in cyclic cows [2]. Furthermore, the decrease in the pre-ovulatory release of LH during heat stress reduced the expression of estrus behavior and delayed ovulation. Also in goats, exposition to high environmental temperatures induced lower follicular fluid and plasma estradiol concentrations and reduced LH receptor levels following lagged ovulation [8]. Estradiol secretion in the ovarian follicle is depressed under heat stress, primarily due to reduced theca cell androstenedione production associated with low 17α-hydroxylase expression. In addition, reduced granulosa cells aromatase activity and viability also contribute to poor estradiol secretion. In the case of dominant follicles, subsequent plasma progesterone concentrations are reduced during heat stress and result in the small size of ovulatory follicles with low tonic LH stimulation of luteinization and steroidogenesis [17]. Moreover, low progesterone secretion limits the endometrial function and subsequent embryo development. The increased level of circulating prolactin leads to suspension of estrous cycles and infertility during heat stress [18–20].

2.2. Follicular growth and development

Heat stress damages the developing follicles whenever the core body temperature exceeds 40°C [9]. Heat stress alters the follicular development by reducing steroid hormone secretion, which disrupts the oocyte growth, reduces the growth of dominant follicles and increased growth of subordinate follicles. Heat stressed lactating Holstein cows present smaller follicular diameter compared to non-stressed cows (14.5 vs. 16.4 mm, respectively) showed and also reduced fluid volume (1.1 vs.1.9 ml, respectively) [21]. In addition, heat stress was associated with reduced follicular dominance by prompting numerous large follicles with diameters above 10 mm, with prolonged dominance of ovulatory follicles [10]. Thus, the selection and dominance of normal follicles could be disturbed by high tonic follicular stimulating hormone (FSH) availability [2]. Low LH and the negative animal energy balance during summer prevent the maturation and ovulation of dominant follicles [17]. As the prolonged follicular dominance disrupts the normal oocyte maturation and reduces their developmental competence, the development of small dominant follicles during higher temperature results in ovulation of the infertile oocyte or subfunctional corpora lutea. The regression of the premature dominant follicle before attaining the larger size leads to a substantial reduction in ovulation percentage [8, 11, 17].

2.3. Effects of heat stress on estrus incidences

The seasonal cycle of reproduction in female animals is primarily controlled by the photoperiod, and it was found to be affected drastically by climate changes. Some studies proved the negative influence of heat stress on estrus incidence and duration and hence on estrus detection [6]. The length and intensity of estrus are inversely associated with the environmental temperatures, with higher temperatures triggering an increase prevalence of anestrus and silent heat in farm animals [18, 22]. A significant reduction in the interestrous interval was reported in Japanese black cattle during summer (21.5 days) compared to winter (23.4 days) [23]. Also, Bulbul and Ataman [24] report a decrease in estrus occurrences in cattle with an ambient temperature above 20.5°C. Likewise, decreased estrus duration and delayed onset of estrus were reported in heat stressed Bharat Merino ewes, which were attributed to abnormal LH pulsatility and lower estrogen synthesis during heat stress condition [25]. Malpura ewes exposed to multiple stresses (heat stress, nutritional stress, and walking stress) recorded lower estrous percentage and estrus duration in compared to control (41.7 vs. 66.67% and 14.4 vs. 32 h, respectively) [26, 27]. Similarly, a lower rate of estrus detection was reported in summer compared to spring and winter in dairy cattle. Contrasting to cattle, buffalos exhibit estrus when the ambient temperature is low, with THI value of less than 70 [1, 28].

In addition to ambient temperature, the humidity and solar irradiation also affected the expression of reproductive rhythm in buffaloes and cattle [29]. A diurnal rhythm of estrus behavior has been observed in the majority of Murrah buffaloes, with 60% of estrus exhibited between 22.00 and 6.00 h [28].

2.4. Sexual behavior

Sexual behavior acts as a core indicator of the reproductive activity in livestock females. It was found to be negatively influenced by environmental stressors like elevated temperature [30]. Reduced sexual behavior is reported in livestock during the hottest parts of the day. Wilson et al. [31] suggested that heat stress inhibits the follicular growth during the pre-ovulatory period of proestrus and reduces the intensity of estrus signs by decreasing the level of estradiol. Heat stress also modifies cow behavior, such as decreased walking time during estrus, which contributes to poor estrus detection in dairy cows during summer compared to winter [22]. Cows are less likely to exhibit standing heat during day time in summer months and often shows estrus at night hours when the ambient temperature is low [32]. Upadhyay et al. [28] reported that the low level of estradiol on the day of estrus also leads to poor expression of heat in Indian buffaloes during the summer period, favoring feeble estrus detection in buffalos during the summer season [29]. In cows, behavioral estrus is markedly reduced in summer, when THI is around 78 [28, 29, 33], while the incidence of anestrus and silent ovulation increases [34]. The cows in estrus mount more frequently during winter compared to summer, when detection of estrus is challenging. Furthermore, Japanese Black cattle exposed to heat stress showed lower locomotor activity during estrus, which was attributed to a reduced estradiol 17β production [23].

2.5. Effect on oocyte competence

Heat stress reduces oocyte developmental competence by affecting growth and maturation through an increase in oxidative damage and apoptotic cell death, as well as by inducing irreversible changes on cytoskeleton and meiotic spindle [10]. The elevated temperature may negatively affect the oocyte growth, protein synthesis and the formation of transcripts required for subsequent embryonic development [35]. Reduced mRNA content and storage protein for early embryonic development along with altered membrane integrity affects signal transduction and protein transport. Therefore, prolonged follicular dominance leads to premature meiosis and aged oocytes with the poor developmental prospect. Incomplete dominance could result in ovulation of an aged follicle containing oocytes with reduced competence. Among other effects, incompetent oocytes become transcriptionally inactive by reaching a diameter of 110 μm and lose the ability to synthesize heat shock protein 70 (HSP70) in response to heat shock [36].

In summer, heat stressed Holstein cows exhibit lower proportion of oocytes and cleaved embryos that could have otherwise developed into blastocysts by day 8 [11]. Oocytes exposed *in vitro* to different temperatures (38.5, 40 and 41°C) showed altered maturation, namely a decreased in the percentage of mature oocytes retrieved when cultured at 40 and 41°C, compared with the proportion obtained during culture at 38.5°C [31]. Oocytes cultured at 41°C arrested their development at metaphase 1 stage [37]. Other *in vitro* experiments demonstrated that under elevated temperature conditions the oocytes evidence a decrease in protein synthesis, disturbed microfilament and microtubule architecture, disorganization of the meiotic spindle and increased incidence of induced cell death due to apoptosis [35]. The protein impairment and the increased production of free radical in oocytes alter the zona pellucida layer and the oocyte cytoplasm which in turn impair sperm penetration. Therefore, reduced oocyte competence and stress induced oocyte lesions in the early stages of follicular growth result in poor fertility rate [2].

However, even though *Bos indicus* cows exhibited reduced oocyte quality during chronic heat exposure, they do not show any significant changes in the oocyte quality or competence during acute heat stress [38, 39]. This suggests that either the animal genetics or the length of heat stress may determine the impact of heat stress in cattle reproduction. Thereby, multifactorial mechanisms are involved in the reduction of fertility of domestic animals during heat stress [6].

2.6. Fertility

The high yielding lactating cows are more adversely affected by heat stress than heifers because of their increased metabolism, which generates greater internal heat production thus lowering their fertility rate in summer and autumn compared to winter periods [36]. Heat stress before insemination has been associated with decreased fertility in cattle and sheep [11]. Fertility decreases in buffaloes exposed to THI above 75 in subtropical climatic condition as compared to cattle, since buffaloes are more sensitive to heat stress [6]. The increase of uterine temperature by 0.5°C during hot days causes a decrease in the rate of fertilization [30] since in severely heat stressed cows most damages over the conceptus occur between estrus and day 7 of pregnancy [39].

Heat stress-related infertility is a current worldwide concern in the livestock industry, particularly in dairy cattle. A report reveals a higher percentage of reduction in conception rate during summer months as compared to cooler months [40]. The elevated environmental temperature on the day of insemination is negatively associated with conception rates [41–43]. Impaired conception was associated with heat stress in livestock, either during the breeding period or 42 days before and 40 days after insemination [42]. The conception rate in high yielding Israeli cows was 45% in winter and 20% in summer [2, 44, 45]. Also, Chebel et al. [46] reported a 20–27% drop in conception rates and a decrease in 90-day non-return rate to the first service in lactating dairy cows during summer. In dairy cows, the percentage of conception rate is reduced by 4.6% for each unit increase in THI above 70 and in practical reality, conception rate was often declined to less than 10% during summer [32, 47].

2.7. Embryonic growth and development

The embryonic loss is another important factor that affects fertility in cattle, and bovine embryos are sensitive to maternal heat stress during the first 2 weeks after breeding [17, 36]. A major source for a reduction in embryonic survival induced by heat stress may be due to the adverse effects of elevated body temperatures on developing zygotes and embryos. High ambient temperatures during oocyte maturation and ovulation or during the first 3–7 day of pregnancy reduced the embryonic viability and development. Although elevated temperatures affect the pre-attachment stage of embryos, the degree of the effect decreases as the embryo develops. Heat stress causes embryonic death by the interfering with protein synthesis, oxidative cell damage, reduction in successful pregnancy recognition and expression of stress-related genes associated with apoptosis. The exposure of lactating cows to heat stress after the 1st day of estrus has reduced the development of embryos to blastocyst stage after 8th day of estrus [39], the deleterious effects of heat stress on the embryos being most evident in early stages of its development [48]. *In vitro* or *in vivo* exposure of embryos to high temperatures until day 7 (blastocyst stage) is accompanied by lower pregnancy rates up to day 30 and higher rates of embryonic loss occurred on day 42 of gestation [48]. Embryos at day 1 are more susceptible to maternal heat stress than embryos at days 3–7. In addition, heat stressed embryo at the time of post-implantation period was found to be associated with foetal malnutrition and various other teratologic conditions in cows, which may ultimately culminate in embryonic death [22].

2.8. Impact on pregnancy

Heat stress negatively affects the ability of an animal to become pregnant through many mechanisms affecting fertilization, follicular development and early embryonic development (**Figure 2**). Ryan et al. [49] reported that when the rectal temperature of the animals increased from 38.5 to 40°C at 72 h after insemination, pregnancy rate decreased up to 50%. Amundson et al. [45] also found a significant reduction in the pregnancy rate in beef cattle during summer (62%) when the THI was equal to or above 72.9. Likewise, Amundson et al. [50] reported

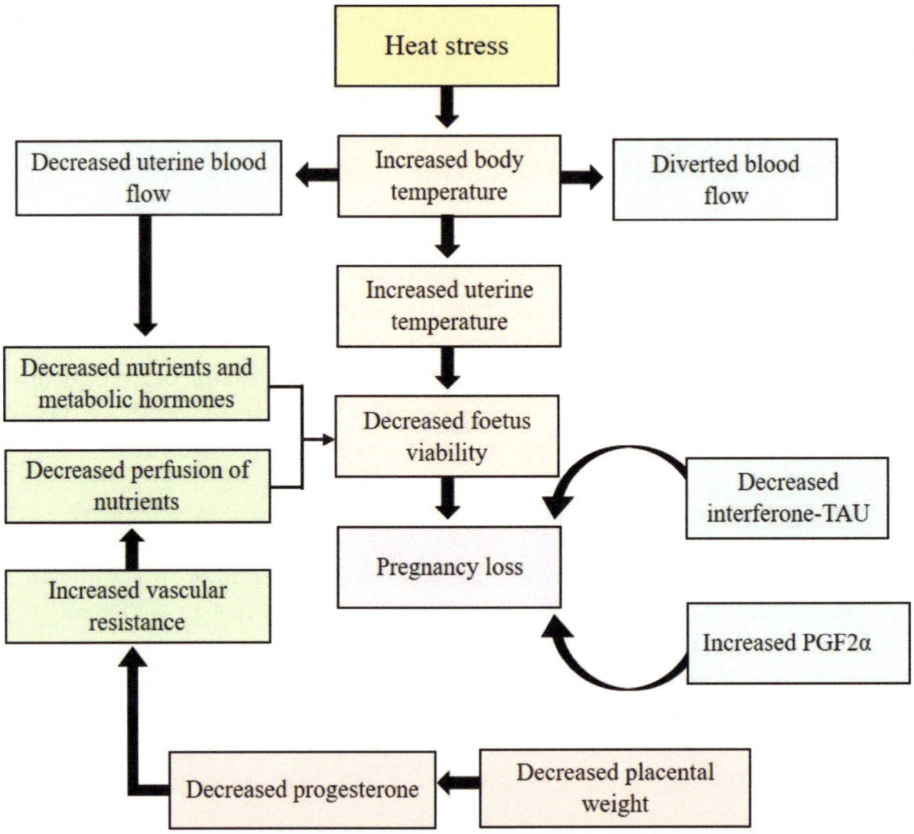

Figure 2. Impact of heat stress on pregnancy in livestock.

3.2% decrease in pregnancy rates in *Bos taurus* cattle for each unit increase in THI above 70, and a decrease of 3.5% for each degree increase in ambient temperature above 23.4°C. Further, heat stress during pregnancy slows down the growth of the foetus, which was attributed to the decreased uterine blood supply [51], which hampers supply of nutrients and hormones to the conceptus [45]. Slow growing embryos fail to signal pregnancy to the maternal organism in due time. Therefore, the endometrial prostaglandin F2alpha (PGF2α) secretion tends to increase during heat stress and trigger luteolysis, thereby threatening the maintenance of pregnancy [29]. Each additional raise of 1.05 unit in the THI over 72, during the peri–implantation period, during 21–30 days and up to 90 days of gestation, increases the chance of pregnancy losses [39]. The placental weight and hormonal secretions are reduced and the vascular resistance is increased during heat stress, which further affects the reduction in perfusion of nutrients to the foetus [23].

2.9. Impact on maternal recognition of pregnancy

The maximum pregnancy losses due to heat stress occur during the early embryonic period of 8–17 days of pregnancy [52, 53]. In addition, heat stress compromises the embryonic growth up to day 17, which was considered a critical period for production of interferon-tau by the embryo. The quantity of interferon-tau is crucial to reduce the pulsatile secretion of PGF2α thus facilitating the persistence of the corpus luteum for the maintenance of pregnancy. Hence, low-quality embryo and poor quality CL are important causes of early embryonic death during heat stress. The heat stress during late gestation period in dairy cows resulted in lower birth weight calves with reduced milk yield, which is associated with a reduced thyroxine, prolactin and growth hormone [54].

2.10. Pre-partum period and days open

The dry period is a critical period, in which the mammary gland involution, the rapid fetal growth and induction of lactation occurs, with subsequent mammary development [36]. Heat stress in the cow impairs the placental hormones secretion, which can negatively affect the intrauterine fetal growth and reduce milk yield [10]. Heat stress in mid to late pregnancy can affect endocrine responses that may increase foetal abortions, shorten the gestation length, lower calf birth weight, and reduce follicular and oocyte maturation in postpartum estrous cycles [55]. Pre-partum heat stress may also decrease thyroid hormones and placental estrogen levels, while increasing non-esterified fatty acid concentrations in blood that alters the growth of the udder and placenta, placental angiogenesis, nutrients supply to the unborn calf and subsequent milk production [10, 54].

The major impact of heat stress on postpartum involves a delay of the return to gestation due to decreased submission rate and low conception/pregnancy rates [55], as already mentioned. Ray et al. [56] reported that first lactation cows are more sensitive to summer stress with the significantly longer postpartum period than cows with multiple lactations. On the other hand, Lewis et al. [57] reported that the heat stress did not alter postpartum days from calving to first estrus, in clear contradiction with Jonsson et al. [58], who suggested that the heat stress induced reduction in dry matter intake may lead to increased negative energy balance, therefore prolonging the postpartum period and reducing the fertility in dairy cows. Further, the negative energy balance decreased the plasma concentrations of insulin and glucose and caused delayed ovulation [33]. The poor folliculogenesis and delayed ovulations during heat stress resulted in longer calving interval, reduced the birth weight and milk yield [51]. Further, longer service period in buffaloes during summer may be due to the higher incidence of silent estrus [1].

3. Male reproductive performance

Bulls are generally considered to be half of the herd and its fertility is directly associated with the fertilization of oocyte to produce a good, viable and genetically potential concepts. In mammalian species, the males have a unique physiological mechanism of testicular thermoregulation to maintain its reproductive activity in adverse environmental conditions [59]. The increased density of sweat glands in the scrotum of ruminants is crucial to the efficiency of local thermoregulation. The testicular temperature in bulls must be 4–5°C below the rectal temperature, and this difference in temperature is essential for an efficient sperm production

[60]. The optimal ambient temperature for efficient sperm production could be approximately 15–20°C. Males are highly susceptible to the pooled effect of high ambient temperature, relative humidity, solar radiation and the wind, and this reduces both the quantity and quality of sperm production, thereby decreasing the male fertility [6, 61] (**Figure 3**). Also, high temperatures interfere with the oxidative metabolism of glucose in spermatic cells as a result of mitochondrial dysfunctions and the accumulation of reactive oxygen species and increase lipid peroxidation which is reflected in an increase of sperm primary defects [62].

The scrotum of bull has thin skin with low fat, low pelage, highly vascularized [59], and its participation in the thermoregulation mechanism is coupled with physical mechanism of counter-current mechanism for heat exchange and blood flow regulation centered in the testicular cord. This complex mechanism allows the maintenance of testicular temperature between 2 and 6°C below body temperature [63]. The local thermoregulation is approbated by relaxation of the dartos (in the scrotum) which together with distension of the cremaster

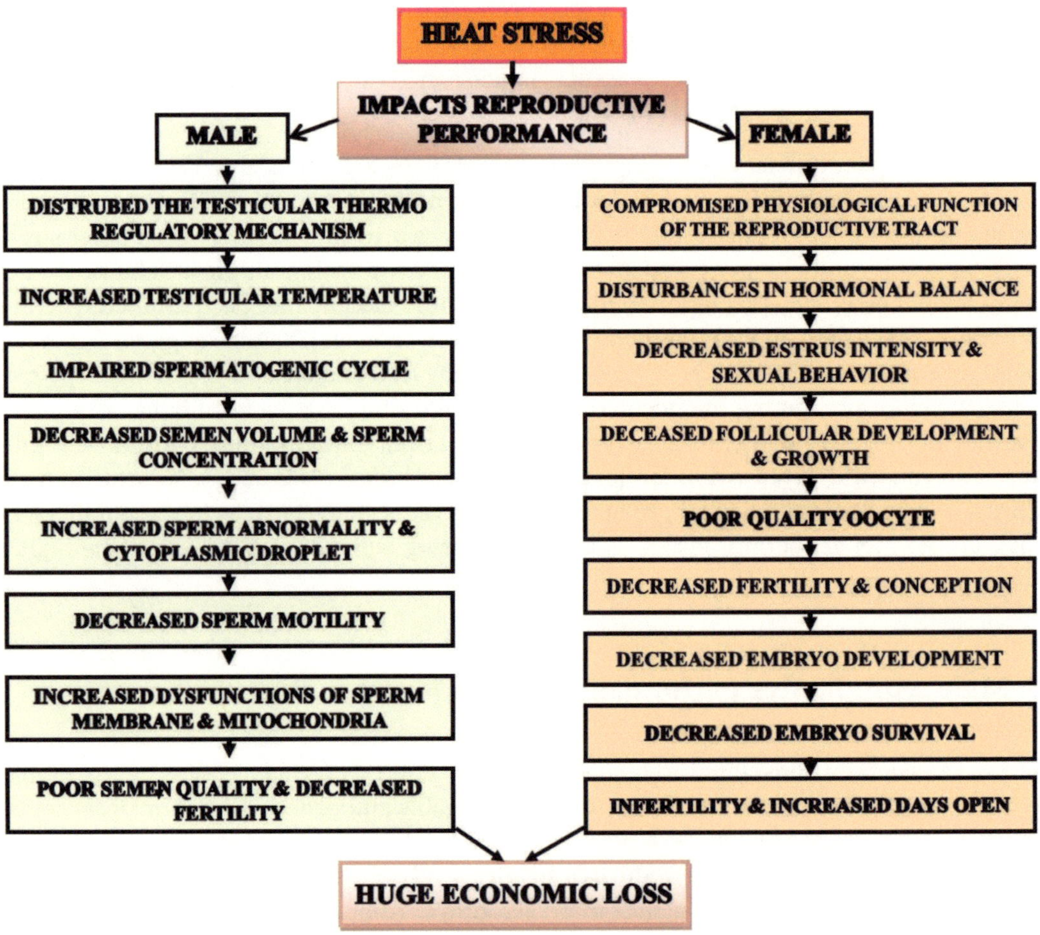

Figure 3. Impact of heat stress on the reproductive performances of livestock.

muscle (in the testicular cord) will increase the distance between the testes and the body cavity [63]. Marai et al. [64] reported that the length of the tunica dartos was greater in summer and autumn than in winter, in rams. Further, it has been established that a high ambient temperature during summer significantly increases the scrotal skin temperature in males. In spite of the efficiency of this mechanism, exposure of the animals to high environmental temperature changes the thermoregulatory mechanisms depending on the thermal gradient and may cause a degeneration of testicular parenchyma which was associated with subfertility and infertility in males, which will negatively impact semen quality and quantity with subsequent reduction in ruminants fertility [63].

The heat stress may also cause a temporary interruption in the semen production, sperm motility and an increase in the sperm secondary defects [65]. Some reports refer that the scrotal skin temperature exhibits highly negative correlation with serum testosterone, libido, sperm motility, sperm concentration and conception rate while it was positively associated with dead and total abnormal sperm [64, 66]. High testicular temperature also results in spermatogonia apoptosis in the seminiferous tubules, degeneration of Sertoli and Leydig cells and disruption of DNA strands, particularly in pachytene spermatocytes and round spermatids [55]. Further, direct exposure of the testes to high temperature also alters the spermatogenic cycle affecting the quality of ejaculate [22]. The changes in libido and sexual behavior in bulls are governed by an imbalance in hypothalamus-hypophyseal-gonadal axis culminating in low testosterone level, sperm output, and motility. In addition, semen attributes like sperm concentration, sperm motility, sperm viability, sperm morphology and acrosome integrity are negatively influenced by heat stress in bulls and bucks, which may ultimately lead to infertility [46, 55].

3.1. Spermatogenesis

The major indicators of sperm production capacity and spermatogenic functions are scrotal circumference and testicular consistency, tone, size and weight that are usually inversely related to higher ambient temperatures. Sahni and Roy [67] reported that the maximum and minimum temperatures for optimum spermatogenesis are 29.4 and 15.6°C, respectively. The elevated temperature hampers the process of spermatogenesis by degeneration of sperm cells and subsequently reduces the fertilizing ability of spermatozoa. Further, seminal characteristics are affected by high temperature and humidity, which affects the spermiogenic phase 18 days before semen collection [68].

Moreover, spermatogenesis is also extremely sensitive to ionizing irradiation and relative humidity above 50% can destroy the proliferating spermatogonia [50]. The analysis of semen obtained from heat stressed bulls showed a reduction in volume and motility along with numerous secondary sperm defects [65]. In addition, the total number of dead and abnormal sperm cells also increased in response to heat stress. The histological sections of testes from heat stressed males showed unchanged or increased interstitium while the spermatogenic elements were seldom found. Further, heat stress was reported to reduce the breeding efficiency in males as the number of testicular cells like secondary spermatocytes and spermatids, the ratio of Sertoli cells to other cells and the diameter of the seminiferous tubules are significantly reduced [35]. Kastelic et al. [69] reported that the minimal temperature gradient between proximal and distal poles of the scrotum in warm periods causes increased sperm damage, mass activity, sperm motility, and vigour. Exposure of the bull to extreme environmental temperature tends to damage the primary spermatocytes, spermatids, and spermatozoa. However, cold stress is likely to be less damaging than higher temperature, and it further was established that the animals during cold stress are able to maintain a scrotal temperature through scrotal thermoregulation [70].

3.2. Semen characteristics

As a consequence of heat stress in males, the biological phenomena such as sexual activity, endocrine secretions and testicular function, spermatogenesis and physical and chemical characteristics of semen are affected. Extremes of environmental temperature may cause low sperm quality, which is closely related to female low fertility, as a result of low fertilization rates and increased embryonic mortality. Abdel-Hafez [71] reported that the reaction time, percentage of sperm abnormalities, dead sperm and acrosomal damage were positively associated with testicular temperature while semen pH, ejaculate volume, sperm motility and sperm concentration ($\times 10^9$ ml) were negatively related. The semen volume, number of spermatozoa and motile sperm cells per ejaculation of bulls are lower in summer than in winter and spring. Nichi et al. [62] reported a higher percentage of major sperm defects during summer than winter in Simmental and Nellore bulls. Conversely, Karagiannidis et al. [72] refer an improvement of semen characteristics of bucks reared in Greece during summer and autumn. The critical temperature for the inhibition of spermatogenesis was established to be around 29.4°C under continuous exposure where the higher temperature can alter the scrotal thermoregulatory mechanism [73].

High temperature can also affect semen production and quality during epididymal maturation or spermatogenesis, not only at the moment of semen collection but up to 70 days before collection. Even though the heat stress has minimal effects on the testicular endocrinology in bulls, the same level of heat stress alters the steroidogenesis in boars [74]. Coulter and Lunstra [75] reported that the percentage of sperm motility was 42% at the temperature gradient of 2–4°C whereas Menegassi et al. [68] reported 53% with a temperature gradient of 0.9°C during summer. The bulls representing an abnormal temperature pattern during heat stress enhanced the percentage of cytoplasmic droplets in sperm cells by 13.4%.

Pigs are very sensitive to hot conditions due to the low sweating capacity. Kunavongkrita et al. [76] reported lower semen volume with less sperm concentration (174×10^6) per mL during summer in comparison with winter (266×10^6) in bulls. The biochemical elements of semen such as fructose, citric acid, and sodium and potassium, total phosphorus and calcium concentration are reduced significantly during heat stress. The semen quality parameters are decreasing with higher lipid peroxidation production as an effect of oxidative stress during summer. The pH of the semen also showed high correlation with environmental temperatures. Further, reduced testosterone concentration was recorded in males exposed to heat stress apart from reducing the reaction time [77].

3.3. Effects of season on semen quality

Sexual behavior, semen quality and quantity are the main factors limiting the male reproductive efficiency in a year. Possible fluctuations in seminal quality are associated with factors such as breed, age, seasonality, temperature, photoperiod and other factors of different etiologies [78]. The month and season of the year show a significant effect on semen quality parameters. The semen output increases when the relative humidity is around 50% and decreases markedly in sperm concentration and total sperm output at temperature of 37°C with 80% relative humidity [79]. The semen volume and sperm concentration are lowest in the summer and gradually increase during the spring and reach a peak in late autumn [78]. Heat stressed bulls produced low quality semen with high number of abnormal heads and cytoplasmic droplets during summer [80]. The seasonal infertility in rams during summer months was attributed to an early occurrence of the acrosome reaction, which could be due to a decreased in acrosomal stabilizing protein in the seminal plasma [55].

4. Mitigation strategies to ameliorate the impact of heat stress

The effects of heat stress on livestock cause huge economic losses to the farmers, but there are few opportunities to recover some of the losses by adapting suitable strategies to mitigate heat stress (**Figure 3**). There are three major key components to sustain the productivity of animals in hot environment: through physical modifications of environment, nutritional management and genetic development of breeds that are less sensitive to heat stress [5]. These strategies may either be used individually or in combination to obtain better results by providing optimum productive environment for farm animals. In addition, summer infertility may also be treated with advanced reproductive technologies comprising gonadotropins, timed artificial insemination and embryo transfer. Strategies that are cost effective and involve indigenous knowledge have the better success rate in adopting those strategies by the farmers.

4.1. Physical modification of environment

In general, livestock environmental management is an emerging area in animal science, which is getting more attention in the era of climatic change, attempting to provide a suitable microclimate to ensure optimum production by preventing the adverse environmental impacts on animal production systems. Primary means of altering the environment may be broadly divided into two categories comprising (i) provision of shade and (ii) evaporative cooling techniques [6]. The environmental modifications such as shade and cooling systems are critical in arid and semi-arid zones during heat stress to maintain milk production, milk component levels, reproductive performance and animal welfare [81]. The basics of providing shade are attributed to the efforts in reducing heat load from direct solar irradiation in livestock. These shading structures could be either natural or artificial. Trees are considered to be the most cost effective methodology to provide shade since they protect from the sun and capture radiation by evaporation of humidity in the leaves. Buffington et al. [82] pointed out that painting of upper part of the shade unit with white color and installing a 2.5 cm thick of isolating material may considerably reduce solar radiation. The height of shades in the corral must be from 3.6 to 4.2 m in order to guarantee reduction in solar radiation. It has been established that shading reduces the incoming radiant heat load by 30% or more and shading of the feed and water also offered production advantages for British and European breeds of cattle [83]. The cooling systems alleviate heat load from livestock by using the principle of evaporation, combining water misting and forced ventilation through use of spray and fans, and are frequently placed inside free-stall barns or under shades in open space corrals. Milk production and reproductive performance of dairy cattle are improved by the use of an evaporative cooling system [84]. Furthermore, the animals that are cooled with sprinklers consume more feed with less quantity of water, which has increased milk, fat, protein and production performance [85]. Fogging and misting systems use fine droplets of water, which are immediately dispersed into the air stream by quick evaporation and cool the surrounding environment.

4.2. Nutritional management of heat stress

Ensuring appropriate nutritional level to the livestock is crucial to optimize livestock production in the changing climatic condition. Importance should be given for providing balanced nutrition to ensure optimum reproduction in animals as the energy balance are closely associated with their fertility [86]. The environmental temperatures are highest in arid and semi-arid regions where the available feed resources are both of low quality and quantity which directly affect the reproductive performance of the livestock species. Combating the heat stress effects on the metabolism is therefore very essential, as animals subjected to mild to severe heat stress needs to be supplemented 7–25% extra maintenance requirements [87]. Therefore, to meet their energy requirements, it is essential to enhance the nutrient density by feeding high quality forage, concentrates and fat supplementations. In addition to the supplementation of low fiber, high protein diet was also found to be helpful by reducing the water requirement for metabolism. Feeding of feed additives stabilizes the distorted rumen environment and also improves the energy utilization [88]. Moreover, fat content in the diet has favorable effects on concentrations of cholesterol, progesterone, rate of synthesis and metabolism of PGF2 α, follicle growth and pregnancy rates in dairy herds [89]. Also, dietary supplements of vitamins, trace elements and minerals can ameliorate the adverse effects of heat stress. Vitamin E and selenium injections reduce the rectal temperature and body weight loss in sheep during summer [19]. Supplementation of inorganic chromium in the feed of buffalo calves reared under high ambient temperature improved heat tolerance and the animal immune status without affecting nutrient intake and growth performance. It was also demonstrated that the adverse effect of heat stress on the productive and reproductive efficiency of Malpura ewes were reversed through mineral mixture and antioxidant supplementation [19]. DiGiacomo et al. [90] also reported that the feeding of betaine, a trimethyl form of glycine, ameliorate heat stress in sheep. Feeding buffers during heat stress is highly beneficial to animals, since buffers assist in the prevention of low rumen pH and rumen acidosis [91]. Also, the addition of common macro minerals Na^+ and K^+ in feed increases dry matter intake and production performance [91]. Inclusion of ascorbic acid in the feed ameliorates, heat stress induced problems like poor immunity, feed intake, weight gain, oxidative stress, body temperature, fertility and semen quality [92]. In addition, supplementation of L-ascorbic acid, both singly and in combination with l-tocopherol acetate, was found to be helpful to heat-stressed layers [92].

4.3. Genetic selection of heat-tolerant breeds

Scientific advances allow improving the environmental modifications and nutritional management in the view of alleviating the impacts of thermal stress on animal performance. However, long-term strategies are foreseen for adaptation to climate change, namely regarding the differences in thermal tolerance existing between livestock breeds, endowed with tools to select thermo-tolerant animals. However, the selective breeding of dairy cows for higher milk production has increased the susceptibility of cows to heat stress by compromising the summer production and reproduction. Furthermore, selection for high milk yield reduced the thermoregulatory range of the dairy cow and resulted in heat stress which has magnified the seasonal depression in fertility [15]. Hence, the identification of heat-tolerant animals within high-producing breeds will be useful only if these animals are able to maintain high productivity and survivability when exposed to heat stress conditions. Cattle with shorter hair, hair of greater diameter and lighter coat color are more adapted to hot environments than those with longer hair coats and darker colors [93]. This phenotype has been characterized in *B. taurus* in tropical environment, and this dominant gene is associated with an increased sweating rate, lower rectal temperature and lower respiratory rate in homozygous cattle under hot conditions [94]. The heat shock protein genes that are associated with thermo-tolerance have been used as markers in the marker-assisted selection breeding program. The association of polymorphisms in heat tolerant genes is reported in various breeds such as HSP90AB1, in Thai native cattle [95], or the HSF1 gene, HSP70 A1 A gene and HSBP1 in Chinese Holstein cattle [96, 97]. In addition to HSPs, there are also other thermo-tolerant genes reported in ruminant livestock species which undergo changes in their expression pattern while subjecting them to heat stress. The other genes of economic importance include ATP1B2, thyroid hormone receptor, interleukins, fibroblast growth factor, protein kinase C, NADH dehydrogenase, phosphofructokinase and glycosyl transferase, among others [6, 97]. However, further detailed studies are required to elucidate the expression pattern of these genes in diversified animal species before they may be considered as biological markers to be used in marker assisted selection program to develop thermo-tolerant breeds, which can produce and reproduce normally.

4.4. Hormonal treatment and assisted reproductive technologies

Hormonal treatments have the potential to minimize the heat stress effects in animals. The administration of GnRH in the early stages of estrus coincides with the endogenous LH surge and improves the conception rate successfully. GnRH agonist or hCG injected on day 5 of the estrous cycle results in ovulation or luteinization of the first wave dominant follicle and forms an accessory corpus luteum (CL) that enhances the plasma progesterone levels to compensate its decrease in chronic heat stress [2, 98]. The timed artificial insemination (AI) program also improves summer fertility when associated with an injection of GnRH to induce a programmed recruitment of the ovulatory follicle. This protocol should be followed by PGF2α injection 7 days later to regress the CL which permits the final maturation of ovulatory follicles. Further, a second dose of GnRH 48 h after PGF2α may induce ovulation and the insemination of cows at 16 h to ensure successful conception [99]. The Ovsynch protocol successfully synchronized the ovulation in buffaloes and increased conception rate when combined with timed AI [100]. El-Tarabany and El-Tarabany [101] reported that the CIDRsynch and Presynch protocols improved the conception and pregnancy rate of Holstein cows under subtropical environmental conditions. Embryo transfer (ET) improves pregnancy rates during summer because embryos are transferred after the time at which they are more sensitive to heat stress. Compared to AI, pregnancy rates in cows exposed to heat stress have been improved by transfer of either frozen or unfrozen embryos produced by superovulation [102].

5. Conclusion

Under the climate change scenario, elevated temperature and relative humidity will definitely impose heat stress on all the species of livestock and will adversely affect their reproductive ability. This chapter discussed in detail the impact of heat stress on both female and male reproductive performance. This chapter also elaborated on ameliorative strategies that should be given consideration to prevent economic losses incurred due to environmental stresses on livestock reproduction. Fortunately, proven strategies exist to mitigate some effects of heat stress on animal reproduction. These include housing animals in facilities that minimize heat stress, use of timed AI protocols to overcome poor estrus detection and implementation of embryo transfer programs to bypass damage to the oocyte and early embryo caused by heat stress. Management alternatives, such as the strategic use of shade, wind protection, sprinklers and ventilation in the summer, also need to be considered to help livestock cope with adverse conditions. In addition to these measures, manipulation of diet energy density and intake may also be beneficial for livestock challenged by environmental conditions. There are also several promising avenues of research that may yield new approaches for enhancing reproduction during heat stress. These include administration of antioxidants and manipulation of the growth axis. Opportunities also exist for manipulating animal genetics to develop an animal that is more resistant to heat stress. Genes in animals exist for regulation of body temperature and for cellular resistance to elevated temperature and identification and incorporation of these genes into heat sensitive breeds in a manner that does not reduce production and reproduction would represent an important achievement.

Author details

Govindan Krishnan[1], Madiajagan Bagath[1], Prathap Pragna[1,2], Mallenahally Kusha Vidya[1,3], Joy Aleena[1,2], Payyanakkal Ravindranathan Archana[1,2], Veerasamy Sejian[1]* and Raghavendra Bhatta[1]

*Address all correspondence to: drsejian@gmail.com

1 ICAR—National Institute of Animal Nutrition and Physiology, Bangalore, Karnataka, India

2 Academy of Climate Change Education and Research, Kerala Agricultural University, Thrissur, Kerala, India

3 Veterinary College, Karnataka Veterinary Animal and Fisheries Sciences University, Bangalore, India

References

[1] Singh SV, Upadhyay RC, Ashutosh, Hooda OK, Vaidya MM. Climate change: impacts on reproductive pattern of cattle and buffaloes. Wayamba Journal of Animal Science. 2011; **8**:199-208

[2] Wolfenson D, Roth Z, Meidan R. Impaired reproduction in heat-stressed cattle: basic and applied aspects. Animal Reproduction Science. 2000; **60**:535-547

[3] Gendelman M, Roth Z. Seasonal effect on germinal vesicle-stage bovine oocytes is further expressed by alterations in transcript levels in the developing embryos associated with reduced developmental competence. Biology of Reproduction. 2012a; **86**(1):1-9

[4] Gendelman M, Roth Z. *In vivo* vs. *In vitro* models for studying the effects of elevated temperature on the GV-stage oocyte, subsequent developmental competence and gene expression. Animal Reproduction Science. 2012b;**134**:125-134

[5] Collier RJ, Dahl GE, VanBaale MJ. Major advances associated with environmental effects on dairy cattle. Journal of Dairy Science. 2006;**89**:1244-1253

[6] Dash S, Chakravarty AK, Singh A, Upadhyay A, Singh M, Yousuf S. Effect of heat stress on reproductive performances of dairy cattle and buffaloes. Veterinary World. 2016;**9**(3):235-244

[7] Gauly M, Bollwein H, Breves G, Brugemann K, Danicke S, Das G, Demeler J, Hansen H, Isselstein J, Knnig S, Loholter M, Martinsohn M, Meyer U, Potthoff M, Sanker C, Schroder B, Wrage N, Meibaum B. Future consequences and challenges for dairy cow production systems arising from climate change in Central Europe. Animal. 2013;**7**:843-859

[8] Ozawa M, Tabayashi D, Latief TA, Shimizu T, Oshima I, Kanai Y. Alterations in follicular dynamics and steroidiogenic abilities induced by heat stress during follicular recruitment in goats. Reproduction. 2005;**129**:621-630

[9] Roth Z, Meidan R, Braw-Tal, Wolfenson D. Immediate and delayed effects of heat stress on follicular development and its association with plasma FSH and inhibin concentration in cows. Journal of Reproduction and Fertility. 2000;**120**:83-90

[10] Hansen PJ. Effects of heat stress on mammalian reproduction. Philosophical Transactions of the Royal Society B. 2009;**364**:3341-3350

[11] Al-Katanani YM, Paula-Lopes FF, Hansen PJ. Effect of season and exposure to heat stress on oocyte competence in Holstein cows. Journal of Dairy Science. 2002;**85**:390-396

[12] Masoumi R, Derensis F. Alterations in reproductive hormones during heat stress in dairy cattle. African Journal of Biotechnology. 2013;**10**(29):5552-5558

[13] Reddy S, Rao KA. Effects of climate change on livestock production and mitigation strategies. International Journal of Innovative Research and Review. 2014;**2**(4):124-144

[14] Naqvi SM, Kumar D, Paul RK, Sejian V. Environmental stresses and livestock reproduction. In: Environmental Stress and Amelioration in Livestock Production. Berlin Heidelberg: Springer; 2012. pp. 97-128

[15] Sejian V, Gaughan JB, Bhatta R, Naqvi SMK. Impact of climate change on livestock productivity. Feedipedia. 2016. http://www.feedipedia.org/sites/default/files/public/BH_026 climate_change_livestock.pdf

[16] Gilad E, Meidan R, Berman A, Graber Y, Wolfenson D. Effect of heat stress on tonic and GnRH-induced gonadotrophin secretion in relation to concentration of oestradiol in plasma of cyclic cows. Journal of Reproduction and Fertility. 1993;**99**(2):315-321

[17] Wakayo BU, Brar PS, Prabhakar S. Review on mechanisms of dairy summer infertility and implications for hormonal intervention. Open Veterinary Journal. 2015;**5**(1):6-10

[18] Singh M, Chaudhari BK, Singh JK, Singh AK, Maurya PK. Effects of thermal load on buffalo reproductive performance during summer season. Journal of Biological Science. 2013;**1**(1):1-8

[19] Alamer M. The role of Prolactin in thermoregulation and water balance during heat stress in domestic animals. Asian Journal of Animal and Veterinary Advances. 2011;**(12)**: 1153-1169

[20] Bridges PJ, Brusie MA, Fortune JE. Elevated temperature (heat stress) in vitro reduces androstenedione and estradiol and increases progesterone secretion by follicular cells from bovine dominant follicles. Domestic Animal Endocrinology. 2005;**29**(3):508-522

[21] Badinga L, Thatcher WW, Diaz T, Drost M, Wolfenson D. Effect of environmental heat stress on follicular development and steroidogenesis in lactating Holstein cows. Theriogenology. 1993;**39**:797-810

[22] Kadokawa H, Sakatani M, Hansen PJ. Perspectives on improvement of reproduction in cattle during heat stress in a future Japan. Animal Science Journal. 2012;**83**:439-445

[23] Sakatani M, Alvarez NV, Takahashi M, Hansen PJ. Consequences of physiological heat shock beginning at the zygote stage on embryonic development and expression of stress response genes in cattle. Journal of Dairy Science. 2012;**95**(6):3080-3091

[24] Bulbul B, Ataman MB. The effect of some seasonal conditions on estrus occurrence in cows. Archiv Tierzucht. 2009;**52**(5):459-465

[25] Maurya VP, Naqvi SMK, Gulyani R, Joshi A, Mittal JP. Effect of thermal stress on sexual behaviour of superovulated Bharat Merino ewes. ASIAN Australasian Journal of Animal Sciences. 2005;**18**(10):1403-1406

[26] Sejian V, Maurya VP, Naqvi SMK. Effect of thermal stress, restricted feeding and combined stresses (thermal stress and restricted feeding) on growth and plasma reproductive hormone levels of Malpura ewes under semi-arid tropical environment. Journal of animal physiology and animal nutrition. 2011;**95**(2):252-258

[27] Sejian V, Singh AK, Sahoo A, Naqvi SMK. Effect of mineral mixture and antioxidant supplementation on growth, reproductive performance and adaptive capability of Malpura ewes subjected to heat stress. Journal of Animal Physiology and Animal Nutrition. 2014;**98**:72-83

[28] Vale WG. Effects of environment on buffalo reproduction. Italian Journal of Animal Science. 2007;**6**(2):130-142

[29] Upadhyay RC, Ashutosh, Singh SV. Impactof climate change on reproductive functions of cattle andbuffalo. In: Aggarwal, PK, Editor. Global Climate Change and Indian Agriculture. New Delhi: ICAR; 2009. pp. 107-110

[30] Alejandro CI, Abel VM, Jaime OP, Pedro SA. Environmental stress effect on animal reproduction. Advances in Dairy Research. 2014;**2**(2):1-4

[31] Wilson SJ, Marion RS, Spain JN, Spiers DE, Keisler DH and Lucy MC. Effects of controlled heat stress on ovarian function of dairy cattle. Journal of Dairy Science. 1998;**81**:2139-2144

[32] West JW. Physiological effects of heat stress on production and reproduction. In: The Proceedings of Tri-State Dairy Nutrition Conference; April 16 and 17, 2002; Grand Wayne Center Fort Wayne, Indiana; 2002. pp. 1-9

[33] Nmez MS, Demurcu E, Turk G, Gur S. Effect of season on some fertility parameters of dairy and beef cows in Elazig Province. Turkish Journal of Veterinary & Animal Sciences. 2005;**29**:821-828

[34] Nebel RL, Jobst SM, Dransfield MBG, Pandolfi SM, Balley TL. Use of radio frequency data communication system, Heat Watch, to describe behavioral estrus in dairy cattle. Journal of Dairy Science. 1997;**80**(1):179

[35] Edwards JL, Hansen PJ. Differential responses of bovine oocytes and preimplantatin embryos to heat shock. Molecular Reproduction and Development. 1997;**46**:138-145

[36] Ahmed A, Tiwari1 RP, Mishra GK, Jena B, Dar MA, Bhat AA. Effect of environmental heat stress on reproduction performance of dairy cows. International Journal of Livestock Research. 2015;**5**(4):10-18. DOI: 10.5455/ijlr.20150421122704

[37] Roth Z, Hansen PJ. Disruption of nuclear maturation and rearrangement of cytoskeletal elements in bovine oocytes exposed to heat shock during maturation. Reproduction. 2005;**129**(2):235-244

[38] Torres-Júnior JR de S, Pires M de FA Pires, de Sá WF, Ferreira A de M, Viana JH, Camargo LS, Ramos AA, Folhadella IM, Polisseni J, de Freitas C, Clemente CA, de Sá Filho MF, Paula-Lopes FF, Baruselli PS. Effect of maternal heat-stress on follicular growth and oocyte competence in *Bos indicus* cattle. Theriogenology. 2008;**69**:155-166

[39] Ealy AD, Drost M, Robinson OW, Britt JH. Developmental changes in embryonic resistance to adverse effects of maternal heat stress in cows. Journal Dairy Science. 1993;**76**: 2899-2905

[40] Cavestany D, El-Wishy AB, Foote RH. Effect of season and high environmental temperature on fertility of Holstein cattle. Journal of Dairy Science. 1985;**68**(6):1471-1478

[41] Nabenishi H, Ohta H, Nishimoto T, Morita T, Ashizawa K, Tsuzuki Y. Effect of the temperature-humidity index on body temperature and conception rate of lactating dairy cows in southwestern Japan. Journal of Reproduction and Development. 2011;**57**(4):450-456

[42] Schuller LK, Burfeind O, Heuwieser W. Impact of heat stress on conception rate of dairy cows in the moderate climate considering different temperature-humidity index thresholds, periods relative to breeding, and heat load indices. Theriogenology. 2014;**81**: 1050-1057

[43] Greer E. Heat stress and reproduction in pigs: its role in seasonal infertility. Recent Advances in Animal Nutrition in Australia. 1983;**7**:216-230

[44] Roman-Ponce H, Thatcher WW, Canton D, Barron DH, Wilcox CJ. Thermal stress effects on uterine blood flow in dairy cows. Journal of Animal Science. 1978;**46**:175-180

[45] Amundson JL, Mader TL, Rasby RJ, Hu QS. Environmental effects on pregnancy rate in beef cattle. Journal of Animal Science. 2006;**84**(12):3415-3420

[46] Chebel RC, Santos JEP, Reynolds JP, Cerri RLA, Juchem SO, Overton M. Factor affecting conception rate after artificial insemination and pregnancy loss in lactating dairy cows. Animal Reproduction Science. 2004;**84**:239-255

[47] Paula-Lopes FF, Lima RS, Risolia PHB, Ispada J, Assumpcao MEOA, Visintin JA. Heat stress induced alteration in bovine oocytes: Functional and cellular aspects. Animal Reproduction. 2012; 9(3):395-403

[48] Demetrio DGB, Santos RM, Demetrio CGB, Vasconcelos JLM. Factors affecting conceptionrates following artificial insemination or embryo transfer inlactating Holstein cows. Journal of Dairy Science. 2007;**90**(11):5073-5082

[49] Ryan DP, Prichard JF, Kopel E, Godke RA. Comparing early mortality in dairy cows during hot and cold seasons of the year. Theriogenology. 1993;**39**:719-737

[50] Amundson JL, Mader TL, Rasby RJ, Hu QS. Temperature and temperature–humidity index effects onpregnancy rate in beef cattle. In: Proceedings of 17th International Congress on Biometeorology. Deutscher Wetterdienst, Offenbach, Germany; 2005

[51] Savasani HH, Padodara RJ, Bhadaniya AR, Kalariya VA, Javia BB, Ghodasara SN, Ribadiya NK. Impact of climate on feeding, production and reproduction of animals. Agricultural Reviews. 2015;**36**(1):26-36

[52] Lopez-Gatius F. Is fertility declining in dairy cattle? A retrospectivestudy in northeastern Spain. Theriogenology. 2003;60:89-99

[53] Inskeep EK, Dailey RA. Embryonic death in cattle. Veterinary Clinics: Food Animal Practice. 2005;**21**:437-461

[54] Avendano-Reyes LFD, Alvarez-Valenzuela A, Correa-Calderon JS, Saucedo-Quintero PH, Robinson, Fadel JG. Effect of cooling Holstein cows during the dry period on postpartum performance under heat stress conditions. Livestock Science. 2006;**105**:198-206

[55] Nardone A, Ronchi B, Lacetera N, Ranieri MS, Bernabucci U. Effects of climate changes on animal production and sustainability of livestock systems. Livestock Science. 2010;**130**(1):57-69

[56] Ray DE, Halbach TJ, Armstrong DV. Season and lactation number effects on milk production and reproduction in dairy cattle in Arizona. Journal of Dairy Science. 1992;**75**: 2976-2983

[57] Lewis GS, Thatcher WW, Bliss EL, Drost M, Collier RJ. Effects of heat stress during pregnancy on postpartum reproductive changes in Holstein cows. Journal of Animal Science. 1984;**58**:174-186

[58] Jonsson NN, McGowan MR, McGuigan K, Davison TM, Hussain AM, Kafi M. Relationship among calving season, heat load, energy balance and postpartum ovulation of dairy cows in a subtropical environment. Animal Reproduction Science. 1997;**47**:15-326

[59] Moreira MK, Rodrigues SA. Influence of seasonality on mammals reproduction. Journal of Zoological Sciences. 2015;**4**(1):43-50

[60] Mishra SR, Kundu AK, Mahapatra APK. Effect of ambient temperature on membrane integrity of spermatozoa in different breeds of bulls. The Bioscan. 2013;**8**(1):181-183

[61] Rahman MB, Kamal MM, Rijsselaere T, Vandaele L, Shamsuddin M, Soom AV. Altered chromatin condensation of heat stressed spermatozoa perturbs the dynamics of DNA methylation reprogramming in the paternal genome after *in vitro* fertilisation in cattle. Reproduction Fertility and Development. 2013;**26**(8):1107-1116

[62] Nichi M, Bols PEJ, Zuche RM, Barnabe VH, Goovaerts IGF, Barnabe RC, Cortada CMN. Seasonal variation in semen quality in *Bos indicus* and *Bos taurus* bulls raised under tropical conditions. Theriogenology. 2006;**66**:822-828

[63] Brito LF, Silva AE, Barbosa RT, Kastelic JP. Testicular thermoregulation in *Bos indicus*, crossbred and *Bostaurus*bulls: relationship with scrotal, testicular vascular cone and testicular morphology, and effects on semen quality and sperm production. Theriogenology. 2004; 61(3):511-528.

[64] Marai IFM, El-Darawany AA, Fadiel A, Abdel-Hafez MAM. Physiological traits as affected by heat stress in sheep. Small Ruminant Research. 2007;**71**:1-12

[65] Pinto ME, de-Alencar-Araripe MA, Alencar AA. Effects of scrotal insulation on testis size and semen criteria in Santa Ines hairy sheep raised in the State of Ceara. Northeast of Brazil Rev. Brasileira Zootec. 2001; **30**(6):1704-1711

[66] Ruediger FR, Chacur MGM, Alves FCPE, Oba E, Ramos AA. Digital infrared thermography of the scrotum, semen quality, serumtestosterone levels in Nellore bulls (*Bostaurusindicus*) and theircorrelation with climatic factors. Ciências Agrárias Londrina. 2016;**37**(1):221-232

[67] Sahni KL, Roy A. A note on summer sterility in Romney Marsh rams under tropical conditions. Indian Journal of Veterinary Science. 1967;**37**:335-338

[68] Menegassi SRO, Barcellos JOJ, Dias EA, Koetz C, Pereira GR, Peripolli V, McManus, Canozzi MEA, Lopes FG. Scrotal infrared digital thermography as a predictor of seasonal effects on sperm traits in Braford bulls. International Journal of Biometeorology. 2015;**9**(3):357-364

[69] Kastelic JP, Cook RB, Pierson RA, Coulter GH. Relationships among scrotal and testicular characteristics, sperm production, and seminal quality in 129 beef bulls. Canadian Journal of Veterinary Research. 2001;**65**(2):111-115

[70] Setchell, BP. Heat and the testis. Journal of Reproduction Fertility. 1998;**114**:179-194

[71] Abdel-Hafez, M.A.M., 2002. Studies on the reproductive performance in sheep [Ph.D. thesis]. Zagazig, Egypt: Faculty of Agriculture, Zagazig University

[72] Karagiannidis A, Varsakeli S, Karatzas G. Characteristics and seasonal variations in the semen of Alpine, Saanen and Damascus goat bucks born and raised in Greece. Theriogenology. 2000;**53**:1285-1293

[73] McDowell RE. Improvement of Livestock Production in Warm Climates. San Francisco: Freeman; 1972. pp. 410-449

[74] Barth AD, Bowman PA. The sequential appearance of sperm abnormalities after scrotal insulation or dexamethasone treatment in bull. Canadian Veterinary Journal. 1994;**34**:93-102

[75] Lunstra DD, Coulter GH. Relationship between scrotal infrared temperature patterns and natural-mating fertility in beef bulls. Journal of Animal Science. 1997;**75**:767-774

[76] Kunavongkrita A, Suriyasomboonb A, LundeheimcN, Hearda TW. Management and sperm production of boars under differing environmental conditions. Theriogenology. 2005;**63**:657-667

[77] Balic IM, Milinkovic ST, Samardzija M, Vince S. Effect of age and environmental factors on semen quality, glutathione peroxidase activity and oxidative parameters in Simmental bulls. Theriogenology. 2012;**78**(2):423-431

[78] Petrocelli H, Batista C, Gosalvez J. Seasonal variation in sperm characteristics of boars in southern Uruguay. Revista Brasileira de Zootecnia. 2015;**44**(1):1-7

[79] Mathevon M, Buhr MM, Dekkers JCM. Environmental, management, and genetic factors affecting semen production in Holstein bulls. Journal of Dairy Science. 1998;**81**:3321-3330

[80] Koivisto MB, Costa MTA, Perri SHV, Vicente WRR. The effect of season on semen characteristics and freezability in *Bos indicus* and *Bos taurus* bulls in the southeastern region of Brazil. Reproduction in Domestic Animals. 2009;**44**:587-592

[81] Brantly S. Mitigating heat stress in cattle. Working Trees Info Sheet. USDA National Agroforestry Service. 2013. http://nac.unl.edu/Working_Trees/infosheets.htm

[82] Buffington DE, Collier RJ, Canton GH. Shade man-agement systems to reduce heat stress for dairy cows in hot, humid climates. Transactions American Society of Agricultural Engineers. 1983;**26**:1798-1803

[83] Slimen IB, Najar T, Ghram A, Dabbebi H, Ben Mrad M. Reactive oxygen species, heat stress and oxidative-induced mitochondrial damage. Internal Journal of Hyperthermia. 2014;**30**(7):513-523

[84] SejianV, Valtorta S, Gallardo M, Singh AK. Ameliorative measures to counteract environmental stresses. In: Sejian V, Naqvi SMK, Ezeji T, Lakritz J, Lal R. (Eds). Environmental Stress and Amelioration in Livestock Production. Germany: Springer-Verlag GMbH Publisher; 2012. pp. 153-180

[85] Igono MO, Johnson HD, Stevens BJ, Krause GF, Shanklin MD. Physiological, productive, and economic benefits of shade, spray, and fan system versus shade for Holstein cows during summer heat. Journal of Dairy Science. 1987;**70**:1069-1079

[86] Sejian V, Samal L, Haque N, Bagath M, Hyder I, Maurya VP, Bhatta R, Ravindra JP, Prasad CS, Lal R. Overview on adaptation, mitigation and amelioration strategies to improve livestock production under the changing climatic scenario. In: Sejian V, Gaughan J, Baumgard L, Prasad CS. (Eds). Climate Change Impact on Livestock: Adaptation and Mitigation. New Delhi, India: Springer-Verlag GMbH Publisher; 2015. pp. 359-398

[87] National Research Council. Effect of Environment on Nutrient Requirement of Domestic Animals. Washington, DC: National Academy Press; 1981

[88] Zimbelman RB, Baumgard LH, Collier RJ. Effect of encapsulated niacin on evaporative heat loss and body temperature in moderately heat-stressed lactating Holstein cows. Journal of Dairy Science. 2010;**93**(6):1986-1997

[89] Staples CR, Burke JM, Thatcher WW. Influence of supplemental fats on reproductive tissues and performance of lactating cows. Journal of Dairy Science. 1998;**81**:856-871

[90] DiGiacomo K, Simpson S, Leury BJ, Dunshea FR. Dietary betaine improves physiological responses in sheep under chronic heat load in a dose dependent manner. Journal of Animal Science. 2015;**90**(3):269-275

[91] Chauhan SS, Celi P, Leury B, Liu F, Dunshea FR. Exhaled breath condensate hydrogen peroxide concentration, a novel biomarker for assessment of oxidative stress in sheep during heat stress. Animal Production science. 2015;**56**(7):1105-1112

[92] Abdin Z, Khatoon A. Heat stress in poultry and the beneficial effects of ascorbic acid (vitamin c) supplementation during periods of heat stress. World's Poultry Science Journal. 2013;**69**:135-152

[93] Bernabucci U, Lacetera N, Baumgard LH, Rhoads RP, Ronchi B, Nardone A. Metabolic and hormonal acclimation to heat stress in domesticated ruminants. International Journal of Animal Bioscience. 2010;**4**(7):1167-1183

[94] Mariasegaram R, Chase CC, Jr Chaparro JX, Olson TA, Brenneman RA, Niedz RP. The slick air coat locus maps to chromosome 20 in Senepol-derived cattle. Animal Genetics. 2007;**38**(1):54-59

[95] Deb R, Sajjanar B, Singh U, Kumar S, Singh R, Sengar G, Sharma A. Effect of heat stress on the expression profile of Hsp90 among Sahiwal (*Bos indicus*) and Frieswal (*Bos indicus* × Bos taurus) breed of cattle. Gene. 2014;**536**:435-440

[96] Li Q, Han J, Du F, Ju Z, Huang J, Wang J, Li R, Wang C, Zhong J. Novel SNPs in HSP70A1A gene and the association of polymorphisms with thermo tolerance traits and tissue specific expression in Chinese Holstein cattle. Molecular Biology Reports. 2011;**38**:2657-2663

[97] Wang Y, Huang J, Xia P, He J, Wang C, Ju Z, Li J, Li R, Zhong J, Li Q. Genetic variations of HSBP1 gene and its effect on thermal performance traits in Chinese Holstein cattle. Molecular Biology Reports. 2013;**40**:3877-3882

[98] Samal L. Heat stress in dairy cows - reproductive problems and control measures. International Journal of Livestock Research. 2013;**3**(3):14-23

[99] Pursley J, Silcox RW, Wiltbank MC. Effect of time of artificial insemination on pregnancy rates, calving rates, pregnancy loss and gender ratio after synchronization of ovulation in lactating dairy cows. Journal of Dairy Science. 1998;**81**:2139-2144

[100] Hoque MN, Talukder AK, Akter M, Shamsuddin M. Evaluation of ovsynch protocols for timed artificial insemination in water buffaloes in Bangladesh. Turkish Journal of Veterinary & Animal Sciences. 2014;**38**:418-424

[101] El-Tarabany MS, El-Tarabany AA. Impact of thermal stress on the efficiency of ovulation synchronization protocols in Holstein cows. Animal Reproduction Science. 2015;**160**:138-145

[102] Stewart BM, Block J, Morelli P, Navarette AE, Amstalden M, Bonilla L, Hansen PJ, Bilby TR. Efficacy of embryo transfer in lactating dairy cows during summer using fresh or vitrified embryos produced in vitro with sexsorted semen. Journal of Dairy Science. 2011;**94**:3437-3445

Chapter 5

Role of Melatonin in Reproductive Seasonality in Buffaloes

Tamer Awad Ramadan

Additional information is available at the end of the chapter

http://dx.doi.org/10.5772/intechopen.69549

Abstract

Buffaloes are characterized by seasonal reproductive activity. Anestrus buffalo heifers and lactating buffaloes were used to study the effect of melatonin treatment on the resumption of ovarian activity during out-of-breeding season. Buffaloes of treated group were injected or implanted with melatonin (18 mg melatonin/50 kg body weight). Using CIDR-eCG protocol preceded with melatonin successfully achieved estrus behavior and induced conception rate during out-of-breeding season. Furthermore, the reproductive performance of buffaloes during out-of-breeding season was clearly improved by melatonin implantation in conjunction with CIDR-eCG protocol due to the luteotrophic effect of melatonin expressed as increasing diameter of CL (corpus luteum) and progesterone concentration. This improvement resulted in greater values of conception rate, in melatonin implanted compared to not implanted buffaloes. Melatonin implantation in anestrus buffalo heifers increased the diameter of largest follicles and melatonin concentration but progesterone and luteinizing hormone (LH) concentrations were decreased. In addition, melatonin implantation in anestrus lactating buffaloes increased the SOD (superoxide dismutase) enzyme activity. Sustained release of exogenous melatonin significantly protects against oxidative stress while increasing beneficial total antioxidant capacity (TAC) concentration in summer-stressed anestrus buffaloes. Melatonin implantation in conjunction with CIDR-eCG protocol successfully improved some blood metabolites, in anestrus buffalo heifers during out-of-breeding season under tropical conditions.

Keywords: melatonin, CIDR, buffalo, reproductive seasonality, ovarian activity, oxidative stress

1. Introduction

Even though buffaloes are able to breed throughout the year in tropical regions, but with distance from the equator they show a seasonal breeding pattern [1, 2], that is determined by melatonin secretion in response to short-day length [3]. In general, reproductive activity of buffaloes is mainly determined by day length, climate (ambient temperature and relative humidity) and nutrition [2]. During summer, poor nutrition coupled with high ambient temperature was implicated with anestrus condition in buffaloes [4]. Heat stress in the hot summer months is an important driver of anestrus in buffalo, whose effects are mediated by increased blood concentrations of prolactin [1], leading to decreased progesterone secretion, and, consequently, extended calving to conception intervals due to repeated breeding and, generally, reduced reproductive performance [5].

In buffalo (*Bubalus bubalis*), reduced sexual activity has been reported as coincident with an increase in ambient temperature and day length [6], in either heifers or mature buffaloes. The proportion of buffaloes exhibiting estrus during the period of short-day length was significantly greater than that in the long-day period (74% versus 26%, respectively) [6]. Also, the conception rates are usually lower between February and August [7], and the number of services per conception are higher in animals calving in summer compared to animals calving at all the other seasons [7]. Decreasing day length may be a stronger determinant of the onset puberty and postpartum ovarian activity, whereas ambient temperature and relative humidity may have relatively lesser impact [8]. Nevertheless, the species physiological characteristics adversely affect buffalo dairy industry and result in a typical seasonal calvings that impair milk supply throughout the year [9].

To overcome seasonality and discipline milk production, it is necessary to implement suitable management schemes, particularly for out-of-season breeding [10]. Hormonal therapies to induce estrus and ovulation in anestrus buffaloes became important breeding strategies to achieve these goals. Hormonal treatments, adapted from other seasonal ruminant species, have been designed to control follicular and luteal functions, to synchronize estrus and ovulation and, more importantly, to eliminate estrus detection by scheduled of timed artificial insemination (TAI).

In deep anestrus buffaloes, out-of-season breeding requests the use of melatonin. Melatonin is a hormone produced and stored in the pineal gland during the day and secreted during the dark, starting after sunset and ending at sunrise. Melatonin controls the reproductive rhythm in diverse ruminant species, like goats and sheep (short-day species), and also in horses (long-day species), especially at higher latitudes [11]. Melatonin-mediated pathways regulate GnRH pulsatibility and, therefore, the activity of the reproductive neuroendocrine axis. It also modulates prolactin secretion by acting on the hypophysis. In addition to melatonin, the concomitant application of estrus/ovulation protocols suggests that controlled internal drug release systems (CIDR) gave better results for anestrus buffaloes [12]. The priming of hypothalamo-hypophysial-gonadal (HHG) axis with adequate amounts of P4 is beneficial for the recovery of reproductive function after calving and, hence, a better display of estrus behavior at the induced estrus [13]. Furthermore, the sufficient priming of endometrium with

P4 might be necessary to enhance the conception rate [14]. Melatonin implantation in conjunction with CIDR-eCG protocol successfully induced estrus behavior and enhanced conception rate in anestrus heifers and anestrus lactating buffaloes during out-of-breeding season under tropical conditions [12, 15].

The objectives of this study were to revise the efficacy of melatonin-based treatments for alleviation of the summer-induced decline in ovarian activity in anestrus heifers and lactating buffaloes and also to evaluate its effects on blood hormonal levels and metabolites concentrations, as well as those of antioxidant enzyme activities, as indicators of sustainability of buffaloes to the expenditure of melatonin treatment for preventing summer-induced decline in ovarian activity in true anestrus buffaloes.

2. Characterization of the buffalo reproductive cycle

The reproductive patterns of an animal are a result of the interaction of the endogenous regulatory mechanisms, mainly endocrine, with environmental signals. This complex interaction may deeply affect the reproductive function, e.g., females suspend cyclic ovarian activity in some periods of the year, or respond to the presence of a dominant individual on the group, or they can ovulate and come into estrus during the non-reproductive season. Bashir (2006) [16] has reported that buffaloes calving in summer (June–August) had a shorter calving interval than those calving in other seasons. The longest calving interval observed in buffaloes was calving in winter (December–January). This means that the buffaloes that had calved just before the onset of their breeding season (October–November) had more chances of getting bred than those calving after passing their breeding season. The buffalo heifers attaining their proper weight just before their breeding season are more likely to get bred than those passing this period and thus, may have lower age at puberty and consequently at calving than those attaining proper weight after this season. Based on this hypothesis, while raising the replacement buffalo heifers, efforts should be made to keep an eye on both critical weight of buffaloes for attaining the age at puberty and also the season in which this weight is attained. In this regard, adjustments in feeding regime may be required to get the critical weight of buffalo heifers just before their breeding season. Because once this breeding season is over, then feeding for accelerated growth may not reduce the age at their puberty and then one has to wait for their next breeding season to see the puberty in the heifers.

The normal interestrous interval in buffaloes may vary from 16 to 28 days, the estrus lasting for 10–20 h during breeding season [17]. The interval between the onset of estrus and LH surge is 1–12 hours and ovulation occurs 18–40 h after the LH surge [18]. The reduced intensity of heat symptoms recorded in buffaloes as compared to cows is possibly associated with lower estradiol levels due to smaller size pre-ovulatory follicles [17], in a mechanism that is further exaggerated by low P4 during luteal phase, a reduced pulsatile LH secretion, growth of ovulatory follicle and low estradiol production during summer months [19].

The stress and adverse environmental factors exert a direct effect on the neuroendocrine set-up, resulting in hyperprolactinemia, reduced pulsatile gonadotrophin secretion, poor follicular maturation and poor estradiol production, thereby culminating in poor heat expression and anestrus [20]. The postpartum anestrus has been differentiated into temporary (less than 150 days) and deep anestrus (more than 150 days), according to the time elapsed between calving and conception [3], or into superficial and deep anestrus based upon the presence or absence of follicular turnover [21].

3. Mechanisms regulating seasonal reproduction in buffaloes

The place of origin and gestation length undoubtedly influence the way in which reproductive seasonality occurs. The natural necessity to coincide calving and weaning with the most suitable time of year represents one of the causes of this 'adaptation' process [22]. This time of year should satisfy the nutritional requirements of the offspring through a period in which etiologic agents (infectious and parasitic) are less aggressive and/or present. Those born under the most favorable conditions have brought about the natural selection of individuals endowed with a more ideal reproductive seasonality that promotes the survival of the species [23].

In domestic animals, spring calving (March–May), which guarantees good availability of forage to offspring in temperate zones occurs whenever reproduction takes place in autumn in species with 5-month gestation (sheep and goats) or in the previous spring in the case of 11- and 12-month gestation (horses and donkeys). The same calving period, therefore, is conditioned by the neuroendocrine system. The reactivation of the reproductive cycle with regard to the length of gestation [short day breeder (negative photoperiod) or long breeder (positive photoperiod)] is therefore controlled.

Researchers in Italy [24] showed that buffaloes displaying stronger seasonality showed high plasma melatonin concentrations 2 hours after sunset, even when they were moved to another farm where other females showed low plasma melatonin concentrations and less sensitivity toward light stimulation [25]. The plasma melatonin concentrations had a repeatability of 0.733 [26]. If the heredity of plasma melatonin turns out to be high, as expected on the base of the high repeatability, the determination of plasma melatonin could be incorporated into genetic selection programmes for buffalo [22]. Lincoln [27] showed that sheep presenting continuous cyclic activity throughout the year retain this characteristic even if living at latitudes where other genotypes were sensitive to the light:dark ratio.

The differences between night and day concentrations of plasma melatonin in March were lower in heifers (5.0 times) than in adult buffaloes (28.3 times) [28]. It has been shown that buffaloes that calve in spring were more adaptable to out-of-breeding-mating strategy [26] and the heifers were less sensitive to the photoperiod [22, 28]. Heifer fertility is not compromised by season [22]. During the summer and when daylight hours are more than the dark, there is an increase in blood prolactin, but contrary to the assertions by Madan [7], buffalo regularly conceive. It is believed that hyperprolactinemia is secondary to hypothyroidism [29] during the warm months. Hypothyroidism exerts a positive feedback on thyroid stimulating hormone and hence on thyrotropin-releasing hormone, which in turn promotes an increase in prolactin [22, 23].

4. Methods to manipulate the out-of-season breeding in buffaloes

In small ruminants, induction of 'out-of-season' estrous cycles may be practiced, enabling spring breeding and, therefore, fall lambing/kidding, resulting in winter production of milk and lambs/kids for the winter markets. Several methods to control the reproduction of small ruminants involve the manipulation of the environmental light (extension of hours of light in a day) [30]. Some others are based on the administration of exogenous hormones that modify the physiologic chain of events involved in the sexual cycle (pharmacologic methods) and ultimately modify the luteal phase of the cycle (progesterone/progestagen and prostaglandins) or the annual pattern of reproduction (melatonin). Synchronization of estrous allows the control and short ending of lambing and kidding, with synchronization of weaning and uniform batching of animals to slaughter; it also allows more efficient use of labor and animal facilities. An appropriate management of reproduction allows ewes and does to breed in the spring to increase the supply of product to the market place on a year-round basis. Pharmaceutical control of reproduction is possible, usually through administration of hormones related to the natural estrous cycle, such as progesterone and/or melatonin [31]. Similar treatments can be used to tame the reproductive cycle in buffaloes.

In buffalo, during the out-of-breeding season (spring and summer), the greater light:dark ratio (long days) suppresses the estrus behavior and the occurrence of ovulation. Anestrus buffaloes have insufficient pulsatile secretion of LH to support the final stages of follicular development, and subsequently, estrus behavior and ovulation do not occur, limiting reproductive efficiency, especially in artificial insemination (AI) programs [32]. Therefore, hormonal therapies to induce estrus and ovulation in anestrus buffaloes became important breeding strategies. These hormonal treatments have been designed to control follicular and luteal functions, to synchronize estrus and ovulation and, more importantly, to eliminate estrus detection by preplanned scheduled of timed artificial insemination (TAI).

In most studies, the success rate was lower when treatment was performed in periods of low breeding activity or during seasonal anestrus, and various modified protocols have been tried to improve pregnancy rates. Among the hormonal therapies developed for cattle, GnRH plus PGF2α-based TAI protocols resulted in a reduced ovulatory response when applied in anestrus buffalo [33]. Also, during the out-of-breeding season, when a high incidence of anestrus is expected, lower pregnancy rates are encountered in buffalo cows synchronized with the Ovsynch protocol for TAI [33]. Recent studies in buffalo have demonstrated that similar pregnancy rates at TAI in both breeding and out-of-breeding seasons can be obtained with the use of progesterone (P4), estradiol (E2) and (eCG)-based protocols [34].

Melatonin implants for subcutaneous application have been commercially available in several countries. These implants have been widely used to advance the breeding season of anestrus ewes and goats. Melatonin implants induce high plasma concentrations of melatonin for 24 h every day, without suppressing the endogenous secretion of the pineal hormone during the night. Thereby, implants cause a short day-like response by lengthening the duration of the melatonin signal [35]. The implants contain 18 mg of melatonin and are designed to maintain high plasma melatonin concentrations for at least 60 days, although most of them continue to release the hormone for longer than 100 days [36].

The mechanisms by which melatonin improves reproductive performance are not fully understood, as the pineal hormone can act at different body sites. Effects at hypothalamus-hypophysis level have been previously mentioned, and an effect at ovary level seems to be consistent, either by reducing atresia during late folliculogenesis to increase ovulation rate [16] or by acting as luteotropic agent [37] to improve fertility. The time of treatment is important to guarantee a good efficacy. Melatonin implants inserted around the summer solstice have been widely used as a means of advancing the out-of-breeding season in buffaloes in areas with high latitude.

In buffalo reproduction, few investigations have been made to clarify a relationship between plasma melatonin concentrations and seasonal reproductive pattern. The Mediterranean buffaloes showing seasonal reproductive trend had highest night-time plasma melatonin concentrations in winter and lowest in summer [24]. In another study carried out on heifers and buffaloes, the melatonin levels showed remarkable differences between seasons. In peak summer because of the shortest night, the lowest plasma melatonin with less persistence of melatonin peak were found, whereas the highest concentrations were noted in early winter corresponding to the start of hypothalamic-hypophysial-ovarian axis (HPO) activity [28]. Moreover, low plasma melatonin was associated with a low seasonal ovulatory activity in buffaloes [24]. This decrease in ovulatory activity during long days happens despite the presence of follicles with ovulatory size (12–14 mm) on the ovaries of nulliparous and pluriparous Mediterranean buffaloes [3, 21].

Melatonin appears to act at hypothalamic sites to increase the release of GnRH pulses by modulating the negative feedback potency of estradiol [38], which acts at hypothalamic and hypophysial loci to reduce luteinizing hormone secretion [39]. The photoperiod modulates KiSS-1 expression via melatonin, strongly suggesting that kisspeptin relays photoperiodic information to the HPO axis. Kisspeptin stimulates LH secretion in a GnRH-dependent manner by increasing GnRH secretion into the hypophysial portal blood [40]. Kisspeptin neurons express estrogen and progesterone receptors [41], which are directly regulated by these steroids in a manner consistent with both positive and negative feedback regulation of pulsatile GnRH secretion [41].

The protocol for melatonin application is simple and less demanding than the traditional treatment of induction-synchronization of estrus using progestogens. Administration of melatonin during anestrus seems to improve the fertility. It has been reported that melatonin implants in buffaloes can improve conception rate [12, 15]. Melatonin treatment in buffalo is necessary to induce cyclicity during anestrus in out-of-breeding season in which evidenced an improvement in conception rate [42, 43]. Ramadan et al. [12, 15] found that melatonin implantation alone did not affect the post-treatment reproductive performance in either anestrus buffalo or lactating buffaloes during out-of-breeding season. On the other hand, combined melatonin and CIDR treatments induced cyclicity and enhanced the reproductive performance of anestrus buffalo heifers and anestrus lactating buffaloes during out-of-breeding season [12, 15] (**Figure 1**).

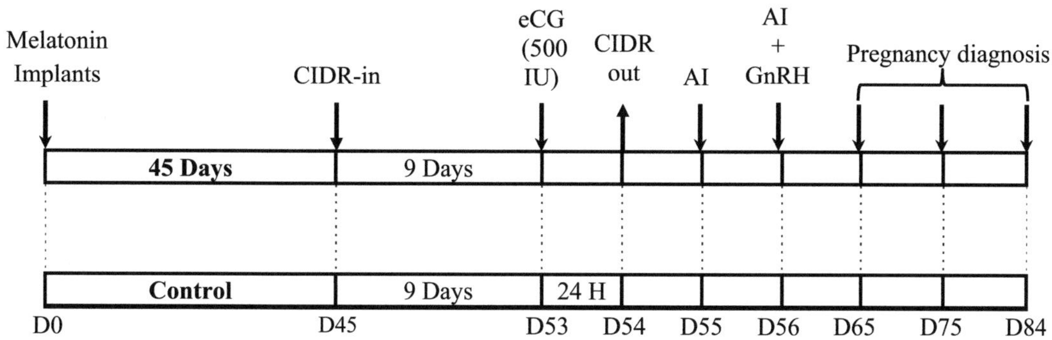

Figure 1. Experimental design to evaluate the effect of melatonin implantation and CIDR-GnRH-based synchronization protocol in heifers and lactating buffaloes. CIDR, controlled internal drug release device (1.38 g progesterone); GnRH, gonadotropin-releasing hormone (10 μg Receptal, i.m); eCG, equine chorionic gonadotropin (500 IU Folligon, i.m) and AI, artificial insemination. Ramadan et al. [12, 15].

5. The effect of exogenous melatonin on hormonal levels and blood metabolites in buffaloes

In anestrus lactating buffaloes injected with melatonin, the serum P4 concentrations increased (0.71 ng/ml) after melatonin injection compared with control group (0.28 ng/ml) at days 12 and 16 post-treatment (post-AI), during the summer season, suggesting a luteotrophic effect of melatonin [42]. Also, exogenous melatonin might improve uterine expression of P4 receptors or their binding capacity, which would result in higher reproductive efficiency [42]. Melatonin implants plus CIDR in buffalo heifers and lactating buffalo were able to maintain the corpus luteum at day 21 of estrous cycle [12, 15]. In addition, the plasma P4 was highest at the second ovulation post-treatment than the first ovulation in implanted anestrus heifers in summer [43] (**Table 1**).

The decrease in P4 concentrations in anestrus lactating buffaloes compared with buffalo heifers was attributed to a prolactin effect. Misztal et al. [44] reported that in lactating ewes the melatonin concentration decreases, whereas prolactin, responsible for the initiation and maintenance of lactation, increases. Prolactin may block the hypothalamic mechanism responsible for episodic release of LH or inhibit the positive feedback of estrogen on LH secretion, and it can even affect ovarian steroidogenesis by altering the number of LH receptors [45].

Lactating buffaloes treated with melatonin alone present higher E_2 concentrations recorded (16 pg/ml) after melatonin treatment in comparison to the control group (9.02 pg/ml) [42]. The pattern of serum E_2 profile in the induced estrous cycle was highest on the day of estrus and decreased in the second week of the cycle [46]. The elevated levels of E_2 4 days before estrus may mediate the LH surge, as demonstrated in cattle [47]. The reducing effect of melatonin on estradiol concentration has also been reported in sheep [38]. Moreover, melatonin decreases the estradiol receptor expression in deep endometrial stroma of ewes, where E2-estradiol receptor complex acts as a luteolytic agent [48]. In ewes, estradiol concentration has also been correlated with the mean response of prostaglandins to oxytocin, via the estrogenic stimulation of uterine oxytocin receptors [49].

Route of administration[1]	Associated treatment	Animal type	P_4 (ng/ml)	E_2 (pg/mL)	LH (mIU/mL)	Melatonin (pg/mL)	Ref(s)
Injection	-	Lactating (n=20)	0.71	16	-	412.3	[42]
Implantation	-	Heifers (n=12)	0.66	-	-	-	[43]
Implantation	CIDR eCG GnRH	Heifers (n=8)	0.72	-	3.44	9.10	[12]
Implantation	CIDR eCG GnRH	Lactating (n=6)	0.97	-	-	6.80	[15]

[1](18 mg/50 kg BW).

CIDR, controlled internal drug release device (1.38 g progesterone); eCG, equine chorionic gonadotropin (500 IU Folligon, i.m at day before CIDR removal) and GnRH, gonadotropin-releasing hormone (10 μg Receptal, i.m at day after CIDR withdrawal).

Table 1. Hormonal levels in anestrus Murrah buffalo before synchronization with melatonin during the non-breeding season.

Melatonin treatment interferes with the effects of melatonin directly in buffalo's hypophysis. In anestrus heifers, with the advancement of melatonin treatment, on days 28 and 42, it resulted in a decrease in serum LH (3.44 mlU/mL) [12]. Melatonin had no effect on the frequency of LH pulses [12]. In sheep, the rise in circulating melatonin is responsible for the increase in GnRH and gonadotropins, thus leading to follicular growth and ovulation [50]. However, this finding is inconsistent with the reduction of LH serum concentration observed in the melatonin-treated buffalo heifers. The failure of high concentrations of serum melatonin to increase LH concentration might be explained by the reduction of buffalo estradiol concentration in summer [51]. Estradiol seems to be positively linked with the action of melatonin on the female reproductive activity, where melatonin exerts a modulatory effect on LH secretion, stimulating its release in the presence of estradiol feedback (cyclic animals) and inhibiting it during steroid deprivation (animals in anestrus) [52]. Also, the presence of low concentrations of plasma GnRH and gonadotropins during the summer period in buffaloes [53] might disturb the development of LH receptors and the synthesis of adequate estradiol in the dominant follicle [51] required to induce the ovulatory surge of gonadotropins [54].

The administration of slow-release melatonin (implants) was responsible for an increase in serum melatonin concentration, ranging from 14.34 to 412.31 pg/ml in treated lactating buffaloes [42]. Administration of exogenous slow-release melatonin induced the restoration of the ovarian activity in summer anestrus buffaloes, which can be explained by a 'cascading effect' of at least a 10-fold increase on the plasma concentrations of GnRH and gonadotrophins, which provides the necessary boost for follicular growth and ovulation [50]. It has been shown that treatments with melatonin implants tend to originate an increase in serum melatonin concentration (9.10 pg/ml) in anestrus buffalo heifers [12] and in anestrus lactating buffalo (6.80 pg/ml) (**Table 1**), which could be associated with the antiprolactinic action of melatonin, as it was suggested in another species [55].

Singh et al. [56] showed that, in anestrus lactating buffalo, melatonin treatments decrease plasma albumin (2.7 g/dl), compared to pre-treatment concentrations. In contrast, Ramadan et al. [57] found higher albumin values (3.41 g/dl) in treated anestrus buffalo heifers implanted with melatonin. Ramadan et al. [57] also reported that the combined treatment of melatonin and CIDR resulted in an increase in plasma concentrations of albumin, glucose, high-density lipoprotein (HDL), alanine aminotransferase (ALT) and reduction in plasma alkaline phosphate (ALP) compared with control animals (**Table 2**). Because of the interaction of melatonin with various endocrine systems [58], it was proposed that melatonin treatment may initiate ovarian cyclicity in true anestrus buffalo heifers through its influence on body metabolism [59]. Albumin, being the most abundant plasma protein, could play a major role as an antioxidant in plasma, mediating thiol oxidation and carbonyl formation [60].

Plasma concentrations of glucose (65.16 mg/dl) were increased by melatonin and CIDR treatment [57]. Glucose is the primary energy source for the ovary and it is possibly metabolized in the ovary through anaerobic pathways. It also stimulates the ovarian follicular growth [61]. Furthermore, plasma glucose is a positive metabolic signal for the central control of GnRH release [62].

Increased lipolysis during lactation is hormonally regulated and not an expression of energy deficiency. Plasma concentrations of HDL (62.29 mg/dl) were increased by melatonin treatment combined with CIDR [57]. The concentration of transaminase enzyme ALT (98.72 IU/L) was increased with treatment of melatonin and CIDR in anestrus buffalo heifers during out-of-season breeding [57]. Singh et al. [56] found that exogenous melatonin did not record any alterations in plasma concentration of AST and ALT enzyme activities in anestrus lactating buffaloes. Thus, minor alterations in AST during treatment period in spite of elevated plasma activities of ALT suggested that hepatic functions were not impaired in the buffalo [63]. Follicular growth is a dynamic process in which follicular development is continuous but accelerates during the later stages of the estrous cycle [64]. Plasma concentrations of ALP (97.99 IU/L) were increased by melatonin treatment combined with CIDR in anestrus buffalo heifers [57]. The ALP content in serum may changes during the estrous cycle [64]. ALP is a lysosomal enzyme that catalyzes various reactions in the body, including synthesis of proteins and DNA turnover within the nucleus [65].

Route of administration[1]	Associated treatment	Animal type	Albumin (g/dl)	Glucose (mg/dl)	HDL (mg/dl)	ALT (IU/L)	ALP (IU/L)	Ref(s)
Implantation	-	Lactating (n=5)	2.7	62.1	35.1	56.4	-	[56]
Implantation	CIDR eCG GnRH	Heifers (n=8)	3.41	65.16	62.29	98.72	97.99	[57]

[1](18 mg/50 kg BW).

CIDR, controlled internal drug release device (1.38 g progesterone); eCG, equine chorionic gonadotropin (500 IU Folligon, i.m at day before CIDR removal); GnRH, gonadotropin-releasing hormone (10 μg Receptal, i.m at day after CIDR withdrawal); HDL, high-density lipoprotein; ALT, alanine aminotransferase and ALP, alkaline phosphate.

Table 2. Serum metabolites and some enzyme activities in anestrus Murrah buffalo synchronized with melatonin during out-of-breeding season.

6. The effect of exogenous melatonin on the antioxidant enzyme activity in buffaloes

Metabolic pressures of adaptation to high milk yield and environmental conditions, especially high ambient temperature, exert a retrograde effect on buffalo reproduction. High temperature-humidity index (THI) predisposes buffaloes to develop oxidative stress [66] with anti-gonadotropic and anti-steroidogenic actions [67]. This in turn is involved in modulation of estrous cycle and uterine environment causing defective embryo development and reproductive failure in buffaloes [68] and also contributes to the elongation of the postpartum anestrus [69]. Jan et al. [70] found that overall greater concentrations of biomarkers of oxidative stress coupled with the reduced concentrations of total antioxidant capacity (TAC) in follicular fluid of acyclic buffaloes are indicative of the involvement of oxidative stress in the suspension of the ovarian activity. Further evidence showed that the oxidative stress and the depletion of the antioxidant activity play a significant role in diminished ovarian function, as evidenced by the significant increment in circulatory malondialdehyde (MDA) and simultaneous decline of TAC in buffalo heifers [71].

Melatonin affects membrane fluidity in different cells under conditions of high oxidative stress, indicating that its mechanism of action relates to possible due to an antioxidant activity associated to the directly scavenging of free radicals and the inhibition of lipid peroxidation [72] and thereby the decrease in MDA concentration. A wide range of antioxidant enzymes are also induced [73], counteracting the generation of free radicals due to inhibition of the activity of some pro-oxidant enzymes such as nitric oxide (NO) synthase and lipoxygenase [72]. Moreover, melatonin stimulates the activity of several enzymes related to the antioxidative defense system [74].

Several authors reported that exogenous melatonin increased blood melatonin level, which has a positive correlation with antioxidant capacity [75]. Kumar et al. [76] refer that the total antioxidant capacity (TAC) in the serum of melatonin-treated female buffalos during summer anestrus tends to be higher (2.22 mmol/L) on days 12 and 24 after the onset of melatonin treatment, compared with the control group (1.42 mmol/L), supporting the previous studies of Ahmed et al. [77]. In the same study [76], it was also shown that the concentrations of serum MDA and NO tend to decrease (3.97 mmol/L and 42.41 mmol/L, respectively) (**Table 3**).

The beneficial effect of a sustained release of melatonin on the increase in TAC and the reduction in MDA and NO concentrations [76] suggests a beneficial effect of melatonin in mitigating the oxidative stress effects on fertility, alike that reported in women [78]. The beneficial effect of exogenous melatonin in the resumption of estrus may be related with the facilitation of cellular functions in the growing follicles, because NO, an important intra-ovarian factor, regulates the process of follicular development through its multifaceted role in angiogenesis, vasodilation, regulation of normal follicular growth and function, steroidogenesis and ovulation [79].

Ramadan et al. [15] observed that melatonin treatment resulted in an increase in blood plasma of SOD (superoxide dismutase, 4.72 U/mg protein) activity in anestrus lactating buffaloes under tropical conditions (**Table 3**). Therefore, the increased activity of erythrocytic SOD in

Route of administration[1]	Associated treatment	Animal type	MDA (μmol/L)	SOD (U/mg protein)	GPx (IU/gHb/m)	Nitric oxide (μmol/L)	TAC (mmol/L)	Ref(s)
Injection	-	Lactating (n=20)	3.97	-	-	42.41	2.22	[76]
Implantation	-	Lactating (n=41)	-	10.14	5.67	-	-	[83]
Implantation	CIDR eCG GnRH	Heifers (n=8)	3.40	4.12	-	-	-	[12]
Implantation	CIDR eCG GnRH	Lactating (n=6)	1.95	4.72	-	-	-	[15]

[1](18 mg/50 kg BW).

CIDR, controlled internal drug release device (1.38 g progesterone); eCG, equine chorionic gonadotropin (500 IU Folligon, i.m at day before CIDR removal); GnRH, gonadotropin-releasing hormone (10 μg Receptal, i.m at day after CIDR withdrawal); MDA, malondialdehyde; SOD, superoxide dismutase; GPx, glutathione peroxidase and TAC, total antioxidant capacity.

Table 3. Antioxidant enzymes, nitric oxide and total antioxidant capacity in anestrus Murrah buffalo synchronized with melatonin during out-of-breeding season.

treated anestrus bovine heifers could be attributed to the physiological upregulation of this enzyme to mitigate superoxide radical challenge [80]. It has been established that, in bovine, the SOD and catalase activities in the CL (corpus luteum) parallel the P4 plasma patterns: the enzymatic activity of catalase and SOD present a sixfold to eightfold increase from day 6 to day 16 of the estrous cycle thereafter decreasing through the luteal regression [80]. SOD plays important roles in the maintenance of luteal function, possibly by rescuing the corpus luteum when pregnancy occurs [81]. It has been reported that SOD acts protectively against superoxide radicals to stimulate P4 production by the corpus luteum [82].

The results of Singh et al. [83] are consistent with the results reported by Kumar et al., in summer anestrus buffaloes [76], which also documented the potential of exogenous melatonin to augment the antioxidative capacity of summer anestrus buffalo [76]. Reactive nitrogen species are another category of potentially destructive substances that react with melatonin. It was suggested that melatonin acts by binding with calmodulin and suppresses the gene transcription of NO synthase enzyme [84]. The enzyme is involved in a rate limiting step in the synthesis of nitric oxide; a known oxidant suggested being a major free radical causing follicular damage, thereby resulting in anovulatory condition in summer anestrus buffalo [84].

7. The effects of exogenous melatonin on the reproductive performance in buffaloes

7.1. Effect of melatonin alone

Estrus response and fertility in melatonin-treated female is largely dependent on the animal status, the association of a progesterone treatment and of animals' management at onset of treatment. According to Kumar et al. [42], a single subcutaneous injection of melatonin

(18 mg/50 kg BW in sterilized corn oil) in summer anestrus water buffalo showed a definite influence on the interval to induced estrus (18 days), obtaining a 90% estrus induction rate. In addition, treatments with melatonin implant (18 mg/50 kg BW) in delayed pubertal buffalo heifers during summer successfully induced estrus within 6–36 days [43]. Also Ghuman et al. [43] reported a successful estrus induction in 100% anestrus buffalo heifers implanted with melatonin in summer season (**Table 4**). However, in other studies on buffalo, melatonin implants alone failed to induce estrus signs for the first 45 days after implantation in either anestrus heifers or lactating buffaloes during summer season [12, 15].

Ghuman et al. [43] showed that melatonin treatment increased the diameter of the largest follicle (14.55 mm) compared to control group (12.2 mm), which might be due to the inability to ovulate even after attaining normal pre-ovulatory diameter (>9 mm) [43]. This suggests that the follicle diameter itself may not be determinant of ovulation. The failure of ovulation of largest follicles could be a drive of a lack of sufficient LH stimulus. The amplitude and frequency of GnRH pulses and, therefore, those of gonadotropins, required to induce the growth of follicles are different from those required for ovulation [85]. The wide extension of the period until estrus induction might be derived from the ovarian structures presented at the ovary at starting of treatment in summer anestrus buffalo heifers. Early responders might have, on the day of melatonin treatment, dominant follicles or follicles emerging in the ovaries, whereas in the later responders the follicles developing in the ovaries still not reached divergence. This hypothesis implies an individual variation in the requirements for exogenous melatonin to attain the threshold level necessary to activate hypothalamus-hypophysial-ovarian axis, as defended by Ghuman et al. [43].

Buffalo heifers in anestrus implanted with melatonin revealed larger CL diameter (15.16 mm) at second ovulation than at first [43]. Ghuman et al. [43] hypothesized that in the absence of a strong negative-feedback effect of estradiol on the hypothalamus, the sustained release of

Route of administration[1]	Associated treatment	Animal type	EIR (day)	Estrus %	LF (mm)	CL (mm)	CR (%)	Ref(s)
Injection	-	Lactating (n=20)	18	90	-	-	-	[76]
Injection	-	Lactating (n=20)	18	90	-	-	32.4	[42]
Implantation	-	Heifers (n=12)	6-36	100	14.55	15.16	-	[43]
Implantation	-	Lactating (n=41)	-	65.8	-	-	-	[83]
Implantation	CIDR eCG GnRH	Heifers (n=8)	-	100	10.04	16.40	37.5	[12]
Implantation	CIDR eCG GnRH	Lactating (n=6)	-	100	13.90	18.33	100	[15]

[1](18 mg/50 kg BW).

CIDR, controlled internal drug release device (1.38 g progesterone); eCG, equine chorionic gonadotropin (500 IU Folligon, i.m at day before CIDR removal); GnRH, gonadotropin-releasing hormone (10 μg Receptal, i.m at day after CIDR withdrawal); EIR, estrus induction response; LF, largest follicle; CL, corpus luteum and CR, conception rate.

Table 4. Estrus response, ovarian activity and conception rate in anestrus Murrah buffalo synchronized with melatonin during out-of-breeding season.

exogenous melatonin in summer anestrus buffalo heifers could stimulate the hypothalamus-hypophysial-ovarian axis triggering the early induction of estrus. Lactating Murrah buffaloes treated with single subcutaneous injection of melatonin during summer evidenced an improvement in conception rate (32.4%) compared to untreated animals (0 %) [42].

7.2. Effect of melatonin plus CIDR

When melatonin treatments are associated to CIDR and eCG, the estrus rate after the progesterone removal recorded 100% in either the buffalo heifers or cows during out-of-breeding season. Also, the diameter of the follicle at the day of AI is higher after melatonin treatment plus CIDR in anestrus heifers and anestrus lactating buffaloes [12, 15]. Moreover, compared to the use of CIDR alone, the association of melatonin treatment and CIDR presented a superior ability to maintain CL for 21 days post-AI (12.5% vs. 37.5 %, respectively) in anestrus heifers or between 21 and 30 days post-AI (33,3% vs. 100 %, respectively) in anestrus lactating buffaloes [12, 15]. The increase in CL size paralleled the increased serum progesterone concentration in either treated buffalo heifers or cows [12, 15] (**Table 4**). Furthermore, melatonin may act directly on the corpus luteum to increase progesterone production [37], instead of decreasing the uterine secretion of prostaglandin F2α [86] or modifying prostaglandin biosynthesis in the hypothalamus [87].

Combined melatonin and CIDR treatments enhanced the reproductive performance of buffalo heifers during out-of-breeding season in comparison with CIDR treatments only [12, 15], which could be explained by the deepness of anestrus. The percentage of conception at day 30 post-AI was threefold higher in the melatonin with CIDR-treated anestrus heifers compared to untreated group (37.5% *vs.* 12.5%) [12], as well as in anestrus lactating buffaloes (100% vs. 33.3%, respectively in the melatonin treated and non-treated groups) [15].

8. Conclusion

So far, it has been believed that milk yield in buffaloes is determined by genetic and environmental factors. In recent years, a special focus has been placed on melatonin treatment on reproductive seasonality. In farm animals, day light changes play a very important role as they establish their yields. The length of day light, and in particular the melatonin profile, is of special importance in buffaloes as they determine reproductive process, in which lactation is the last stage of reproductive physiology. Experiments carried out in buffaloes demonstrated that buffaloes are characterized by seasonal reproductive activity. They become sexually active in response to a decreasing day length in late summer to early autumn. During the out-of-breeding season, buffaloes often exhibit anestrus, which extends the calving to conception interval and, consequently, reduces reproductive performance resulting in seasonal calving and a dramatic disturbance to milk supply throughout the year. To avoid seasonality-related constraints, it is necessary to implement management schemes to overcome reproductive seasonality and regulate production of milk throughout the year. Thus, hormonal therapies to induce estrus and ovulation in anestrus buffaloes are important strategies to overcome seasonality. These hormonal treatments have been designed to control follicular and luteal functions synchronizing estrus and ovulation and, more importantly, to eliminate estrus detection by preplanned scheduled of timed artificial insemination. Melatonin implantation in conjunction with CIDR-eCG protocol successfully induced estrus behavior and enhanced conception rate in anestrus heifers and anestrus lactating buffaloes during out-of-breeding season under tropical conditions.

Author details

Tamer Awad Ramadan

Address all correspondence to: tamereweda1174@yahoo.com

Animal Production Research Institute, Agricultural Research Center, Giza, Egypt

References

[1] Perera BMAO. Reproductive cycles of buffalo. Animal of Reproduction Science. 2011; **124**:194-199. DOI: 10.1016/j.anireprosci.2010.08.022

[2] Singh J, Nanda AS, Adams GP. The reproductive pattern and efficiency of female buffaloes. Animal of Reproduction Science. 2000;**60-61**:593-604. DOI: 10.1016/s0378-4320(00)00109-3

[3] Zicarelli L. Reproductive seasonality in buffalo. In: Proceedings of Third Course on Biotechnology of Reproduction in Buffaloes, Caserta, Italy; 6-10 October, (Issue II). 1997;. p. 29-52

[4] Shah SNH. Comparative studies of seasonal influence on breeding behaviour and conception rate of dairy buffalo and zebu cattle. In: Proceedings 11th International Congress on Animal Reproduction and Artificial Insemination. Book of congress, Dublin, Ireland. 1988;**3**:538-542.

[5] Zicarelli L. Can we consider buffalo a non-precocious and hypofertile species? Italian Journal of Animal Science. 2007;**6**:143-154. DOI: 10.4081/ijas.2007.s2.143

[6] Tailor SP, Jain LS, Gupta HK, Bhatia JS. Oestrus and conception rates in buffaloes under village conditions. Indian Journal Animal Science. 1990;**60**:1020-1021

[7] Madan ML. Status of reproduction in female buffalo. In: Proc. Second World Buffalo congress, Buffalo Production and Health: a compendium of latest research information based on Indian studies. New Delhi, India: ICAR Publication; 1988;**3**(12-16): pp. 89-100

[8] Singh R. Studies on the onset of postpartum ovarian activity in relation to climatic and nutritional status in buffaloes. MVSc thesis. India: Punjab Agriculture, University of Ludhiana; 1993

[9] Neglia G, Gasparrini B, Caracciolo di Brienza V, Di Palo R, Zicarelli L. First pregnancies carried to term after transfer of vitrified buffalo embryos entirely produced in vitro. Veterinary Research Communication. 2004;**1**:233-236. DOI: 10.1023/b:verc.0000045414.65331.6a

[10] Zicarelli L. Enhancing reproductive performance in domestic dairy water buffalo (Bubalus bubalis). In: Lucy MC, Pate JL, Smith MF, Spencer TE, editors. Eighth International Symposium on Reproduction in Domestic Ruminants. Anchorage, Alaska: Nottingham University Press; 2010. p. 443-455. DOI: 10.7313/upo9781907284991.034

[11] Chemineau P, Malpaux B, Delgadillo JA. Control of sheep and goat reproduction: use of light and melatonin. Animal of Reproduction Science. 1992;**30**:157-184. DOI: 10.1016/0378-4320(92)90010-B

[12] Ramadan TA, Sharma RK, Phulia SK, Balhara AK, Ghuman SS, Singh I. Effectiveness of melatonin and controlled internal drug release device treatment on reproductive performance of buffalo heifers during out-of-breeding season under tropical conditions. Theriogenology. 2014;**82**:1296-1302. DOI: 10.1016/j.theriogenology.2014.08.014

[13] De Rensis F, Ronci G, Guarneri P, Nguyen BX, Presicce GA, Huszenicza G, Scaramuzzi RJ. Conception rate after fixed time insemination following ovsynch protocol with and without progesterone supplementation in cyclic and non-cyclic Mediterranean Italian buffaloes (*Bubalus bubalis*). Theriogenology. 2005;**63**:1824-1831. DOI: 10.1016/j.theriogenology.2004.07.024

[14] Stevenson JS, Pursley JR, Garverick HA, Fricke PM, Kesler DJ, Ottobre JS, Wiltbank MC. Treatment of cycling and non-cycling lactating dairy cows with progesterone during ovsynch. Journal of Dairy Science. 2006;**89**:2567-2578. DOI: 10.3168/jds.s0022-0302(06)72333-5

[15] Ramadan TA, Sharma RK, Phulia SK, Balhara AK, Ghuman SS, Singh I. Manipulation of reproductive performance of lactating buffaloes using melatonin and controlled internal drug release device treatment during out-of-breeding season under tropical conditions. Theriogenology. 2016;**86**:1048-1053. DOI: 10.1016/j.theriogenology.2016.03.034

[16] Bashir MK. Genetic and phenotypic aspects of some performance traits of Nili-Ravi buffaloes in Pakistan. PhD Thesis. Univ. Agri., Faisalabad, Pakistan; 2006

[17] Baruselli PS, Mucciolo RG, Vistin JA, Viana WG, Arruda RP, Maduriera EH, Oliveira CA, Molero- Filho JR. Ovarian follicular dynamics during estrus cycle in buffalo. Theriogenology. 1997;**47**:1531-1547. DOI: 10.1016/s0093-691x(97)00159-3

[18] Prakash BS, Sarkar M, Paul Vijay Mishra DP, Mishra A, Meyer HHD. Postpartum endocrinology and prospects for fertility improvement in the lactating riverine buffalo (*Bubalus bubalis*) abd yak (*Poephagus grunniens* L.). Livestock Science. 2005;**98**:13-23. DOI: 10.1016/j.livprodsci.2005.10.014

[19] Awasthi MK, Khare A, Kavani FS, Siddiquee GM, Panchal MT, Shah RR. Is one-wave follicular growth during the estrous cycle a usual phenomenon in water buffaloes (*Bubalus bubalis*). Animal of Reproduction Science. 2006;**92**:241-253. DOI: 10.1016/j.anireprosci.2005.05.024

[20] Phogat JB, Smith RF, Dobson H. The influence of stress on neuroendocrine control of the hypothalamic-pituitary-ovarian axis—A review. Veterinary Bulletin. 1997;**67**:551-567

[21] Presicce GA, Senatore EM, De Santis G, Bella A. Follicle turnover and pregnancy rates following oestrus synchronization protocols in Mediterranean Italian buffaloes (*Bubalus bubalis*). Reproduction in Domestic Animals. 2005;**40**:443-447. DOI: 10.1111/j.1439-0531.2005.00606.x

[22] Zicarelli L, Campanile G, Esposito L, Di Palo R, Boni R, Spadetta M, Montemurro N, Pacelli C, Borghese A, Barile VL, Terzano GM, Annicchiarico G, Allegrini S, De Benedetti A, Malfatti A, Lucaroni A, Todini L Anaestro e induzione dell'estro in bufale acicliche, (Anoestrus and oestrus induction in acyclic buffaloes), Agriculture Ricerca. 1994;**153**:25-40

[23] Zicarelli L, Esposito L, Campanile G, Di Palo R, Armstrong DT. Effect of using vasectomized bulls in A.I. practice on the reproductive efficiency of Italian buffalo cows. Animal Reproduction Science. 1997;**47**:171-180. DOI: 10.1016/s0378-4320(97)00008-0

[24] Parmeggiani A, Di Palo R. Melatonina e stagionalità riproduttiva della bufala. Atti Conv. su "Miglioramento dell'efficienza produttiva e riproduttiva della specie bufalina" Agricolture e Ricerca. 1994;**153**:41-48

[25] Di Palo R, Parmeggiani A, Spadetta M, Campanile G, Esposito L, Seren E, Zicarelli L. Influence of changing farm on the repeatability of melatonin plasma level in Italian Mediterranean buffalo. In: Proceedings of the Fifth World Buffalo Congress, Caserta, Italy. 1997; p. 758-761

[26] Di Palo R, Parmeggiani A, Campanile G, Zicarelli L. Repeatability of melatonin plasma levels in buffaloes bred in Italy. Atti della Societa Italiana delle Scienze Veterinarie. 1993;**47**:331-335

[27] Lincoln GA. Photoperiod-pineal-hypothalamic relay in sheep. Animal Reproduction Science. 1992;**28**:203-217. DOI: 10.1016/0378-4320(92)90107-o

[28] Borghese A, Barile VL, Terzano GM, Pilla AM, Parmeggiani A. Melatonin trend during season in heifers and buffalo cow. Bubalus bubalis 1995;**1**:61-64

[29] Campanile G, Avallone L, d'Angelo A, Di Palo R, Di Meo C. Influence of the season and of the number of days after calving on the pattern of thyroid hormones in buffalo cows. In: Proceedings of the Fourth World Buffalo Congress, São Paulo, Brazil, June. 1994; p. 564-566

[30] Vesely JA. Induction of lambing every eight months in two breeds of sheep by light control with or without hormonal treatment. Animal Production. 1975;**21**:165-174. DOI: 10.1017/s0003356100030580

[31] Abecia J A, Forcada F, González-Bulnes A. Pharmaceutical Control of Reproduction in Sheep and Goats. Veterinary Clinics of North America: Food Animal Practice. 2011;**27**:67-79. DOI: 10.1016/j.cvfa.2010.10.001

[32] Carvalho NAT, Julia GS, Pietro SB. Strategies to overcome seasonal anestrus in water buffalo. Theriogenology. 2016;**86**:200-206. DOI: 10.1016/j.theriogenology.2016.04.032

[33] Souza DC, Carvalho NAT, Soares JG, Monteiro BM, Madureira EH, Baruselli PS. Effect of the presence of corpus luteum in lactating buffaloes on the response to the ovsynch

protocol during the breeding season (preliminary results). 29th Annual Meeting of the Brazilian Embryo Technology Society (SBTE). Gramado, RS, Brazil: Animal Reproduction. 2015; p. 629

[34] Carvalho NAT, Soares JG, Porto Filho RM, Gimenes LU, Souza DC, Nichi M, et al. Equine chorionic gonadotropin improves the efficacy of a timed artificial insemination protocol in buffalo during the nonbreeding season. Theriogenology. 2013;**79**:423-428. DOI: 10.1016/j.theriogenology.2012.10.013

[35] Malpaux B, Viguié C, Skinner DC, et al. Control of the circannual rhythm of reproduction by melatonin in the ewe. Brain Research Bulletin. 1997;**44**:431-438. DOI: 10.1016/s0361-9230(97)00223-2

[36] Forcada F, Abecia JA, Zúñiga O, et al. Variation in the ability of melatonin implants inserted at two different times after the winter solstice to restore reproductive activity in reduced seasonality ewes. Australian Journal of Agricultural Research. 2002;**53**:167-173. DOI: 10.1071/ar00172

[37] Abecia J, Forcada F, Zuñiga O. The effect of melatonin on the secretion of progesterone in sheep and on the development of ovine embryos in vitro. Veterinary Research Communications. 2002;**26**:151-158. DOI:10.1023/a:1014099719034

[38] Noël B, Mandiki S, Perrad B, Bister J, Paquay R. Terminal follicular growth, ovulation rate and hormonal secretion after melatonin pretreatment prior to FGA-PMSG synchronisation in Suffolk ewes at the onset of the breeding season. Small Ruminant Research. 1999;**32**:269-277. DOI:10.1016/s0921-4488(98)00187-4

[39] Caraty A, Locatelli A, Martin G. Biphasic response in the secretion of gonadotrophin releasing hormone in ovariectomized ewes injected with oestradiol. Journal of Endocrinology. 1989;**123**:375-382. DOI:10.1677/joe.0.1230375

[40] Smith JT, Li Q, Yap KS, Shahab M, Roseweir AK, et al. Kisspeptin is essential for the full preovulatory LH surge and stimulates GnRH release from the isolated ovine median eminence. Endocrinology. 2011;**152**:1001-1012. DOI: 10.1210/en.2007-0554

[41] Smith JT, Clay CM, Caraty A, Clarke IJ. KiSS-1 messenger ribonucleic acid expression in the hypothalamus of the ewe is regulated by sex steroids and season. Endocrinology. 2007;**148**:1150-1157. DOI: 10.1210/en.2006-1435

[42] Kumar A, Mehrotra S, Singh G, Maurya VP, Narayanan K, Mahla AS, Chaudhari RK, Singh M, Soni YK, Kumawat BL, Dabas SK, Srivastava N. Supplementation of slow-release melatonin improves recovery of ovarian cyclicity and conception in summer anoestrous buffaloes (*Bubalus bubalis*). Reproduction in Domestic Animals. 2016;**51**:10-17 DOI: 10.1111/rda.12639

[43] Ghuman SS, Singh J, Honparkhe M, Dadarwal D, Dhaliwal GS, Jain AK. Induction of ovulation of ovulatory size non-ovulatory follicles and initiation of ovarian cyclicity in summer anoestrous buffalo heifers (*Bubalus bubalis*) using melatonin implants. Reproduction in Domestic Animals. 2010;**45**:600-607. DOI: 10.1111/j.1439-0531.2008.01310.x

[44] Misztal T, Romanowicz K, Barcikowski B. Natural and melatonin stimulated changes in the circadian rhythm of prolactin secretion in the ewe during seasonal anestrus. Neuroendocrinology. 1997;**66**:360-367. DOI:10.1159/000127259

[45] Sheth A, Wadadekar K, Moodbidri S, Janakiraman K, Paramesh M. 1978. Seasonal alteration in the serum prolactin and LH levels in the water buffaloes. Current Science. 47:75-77.

[46] Arunji JTK. Non-invasive monitoring of buffalo estrous cycle. M.V. Sc. Thesis Submitted to Deemed to be University IVRI, Izatnagar 2008.

[47] Echternkamp SE, Hansel W. Concurrent changes in bovine plasma hormone levels prior to and during the first postpartum estrous cycle. Journal of Animal Science. 1973;**37**:1362-1370. DOI: 10.2527/jas1973.3761362x

[48] Vázquez M, Forcada F, Sosa C, Casao A, Sartore I, Fernández-Foren A, Meikle A, Abecia J. Effect of exogenous melatonin on embryo viability and uterine environment in undernourished ewes. Animal Reproduction Science. 2013;**141**:52-61. DOI:10.1016/j.anireprosci.2013.07.007

[49] Beard A, Lamming G. Oestradiol concentration and the development of the uterine oxytocin receptor and oxytocin-induced PGF2a release in ewes. Reproduction. 1994;**100**:469-475. DOI:10.1530/jrf.0.1000469

[50] Misztal T, Romanowicz K, Barcikowski B. Melatonin–a modulator of the GnRH/LH axis in sheep. Reproduction Biology. 2002a;**2**:267-275

[51] Rao LV, Pandey RS. Seasonal variations in oestradiol-17b and luteinizing hormone in blood of buffalo cows (Bubalus bubalis). Journal Endocrinology. 1983;**98**:251-255. DOI: 10.1677/joe.0.0980251

[52] Misztal T, Romanowicz K, Barcikowski B. Effect of melatonin on daily LH secretion in intact and ovariectomized ewes during the breeding season. Animal Reproduction Science. 2002b;**69**:187-198. DOI: 10.1016/s0378-4320(01)00194-4

[53] Palta P, Madan ML. Alterations in hypophysial responsiveness to synthetic GnRH at different postpartum intervals in Murrah buffalo (*Bubalus bubalis*). Theriogenology. 1995;**44**:403-411. DOI: 10.1016/0093-691x(95)00194-d

[54] Alam MGS, Dobson H. Pituitary responses to a challenge test of GnRH and oestradiol benzoate in postpartum and regularly cycling cows. Animal Reproduction Science. 1987;**14**:1-9. DOI: 10.1016/0378-4320(87)90071-6

[55] Dholpuria S, Vyas S, Purohit GN, Pathak KML. Sonographic monitoring of early follicle growth induced by melatonin implants in camels and the subsequent fertility. Journal of Ultrasound. 2012;**15**:135-141. DOI: 10.1016/j.jus.2012.02.008

[56] Singh J, Ghuman SPS, Dadarwal D, Honparkhe M, Dhaliwal GS, Jain AK. Estimations of blood plasma metabolites following melatonin implants treatment for initiation of ovarian cyclicity in true anestrus buffalo heifers. Indian Journal Animal Science. 2010;**80**:229-231

[57] Ramadan TA, Sharma RK, Phulia SK, Balhara AK, Ghuman SS, Singh I. Effects of melatonin and controlled internal drug release device treatment on blood metabolites of buffalo heifers during out-of-breeding season under tropical conditions. Egyptian Journal of Animal Production. 2015;**52**(Suppl Issue): 9-17

[58] Zieba DA, Klocek B, Williams GL, Romanowicz K, Boliglowa L, Wozniak M. In vitro evidence that leptin suppresses melatonin secretion during long days and stimulates its secretion during short days in seasonal breeding ewe. Domestic Animal Endocrinology. 2007;**33**:358-365. DOI: 10.1016/j.domaniend.2006.06.004

[59] Darul K, Kruczynska H. Effect of melatonin on biochemical variables of the blood in dairy cows. Acta Veterinaria Hungarica. 2004;**52**:361-370. DOI: 10.1556/avet.52.2004.3.11

[60] Himmelfarb J, Mcmonagle E. Albumin is the major plasma protein target of oxidant stress in uremia. Kidney International. 2001;**60**:358-363. DOI: 10.1046/j.1523-1755.2001.00807.x

[61] Rabiee AR, Lean IJ, Gooden JM, Miller BG, Scaramuzzi RJ. An evaluation of transovarian uptake of metabolites using arteriovenous differences methods in dairy cattle. Animal Reproduction Science. 1997;**48**:9-25. DOI: 10.1016/s0378-4320(97)00032-8

[62] Foster DL, Nagatani S. Physiological perspectives on leptin as a regulator of reproduction: Role in timing puberty. Biology of Reproduction. 1999;**60**:205-215. DOI: 10.1095/biolreprod60.2.205

[63] Randhawa SS, Uppal SK, Randhawa CS, Brar RS, Joshi BP. Haemato-biochemical profile of buffaloes (*Bubalus bubalis*) with leucoderma. Indian Journal Animal Science. 2009;**79**:12-14

[64] Wise T. Biochemical analysis of bovine follicular fluid: albumin, total protein, lysosomal enzymes, ions, steroids and ascorbic acid content in relation to follicular size, rank, atresia classification and day of estrous cycle. Journal of Animal Science. 1987;**64**:1153-1169. DOI: 10.2527/jas1987.6441153x

[65] Mishra OP, Pandey JN, Gawande PG. Study on biochemical constituents of caprine ovarian follicular fluid after superovulation. Asian Australian Journal Animal Science. 2003;**16**:1711-1715. DOI: 10.5713/ajas.2003.1711

[66] Tucker CB, Rogers AR, Schutz KE. Effect of solar radiation on dairy cattle behaviour, use of shade and body temperature in a pasture-based system. Applied Animal Behaviour Science. 2008;**109**:141-154. DOI: 10.1016/j.applanim.2007.03.015

[67] Shimamura K, Sugino N, Yoshida Y, Nakamura Y, Ogino K, Kate H. Changes in lipid peroxide and antioxidant enzyme activities in corpora lutea during pseudopregnancy in rats. Journal of Reproduction Fertility. 1995;**105**:253-257. DOI: 10.1530/jrf.0.1050253

[68] Khan FA, Das GK. Follicular characteristics and intrafollicular concentrations of nitric oxide and ascorbic acid during ovarian acyclicity in water buffalo (*Bubalus bubalis*). Tropical Animal Health and Production. 2012;**44**:125-131. DOI: 10.1007/s11250-011-9898-x

[69] Megahed GA, Alghandour SEM, Othman RH, El-Zohery FA. The relationship between oxidant/antioxidant imbalance and postpartum fertility in cattle. Assiut Veterinary Medical Journal. 2006;**52**:226-240

[70] Jan MH, Das GK, Khan FA, Singh J, Bashir ST, Khan S, et al. Evaluation of follicular oxidant-antioxidant balance and oxidative damage during reproductive acyclicity in water buffalo (*Bubalus bubalis*). Asian Pacific Journal of Reproduction. 2014;**3**:35-40. DOI: 10.1016/s2305-0500(13)60182-7

[71] Ahmed WM, Bashandy MM, Ibrahim AK, Shalaby SIA, El-Moez SIA, El-Moghazy FM, et al. Investigations on delayed puberty in Egyptian buffalo-heifers with emphasis on clinicopathological changes and treatment using GnRH (Receptal). Global Veterinaria. 2010;**4**:78-85

[72] Reiter J, Tan DX, Manchester LC, Qi W. Biochemical reactivity of melatonin with reactive oxygen and nitrogen species: A review of the evidence. Cell Biochemistry and Biophysics. 2001;**34**:247-256

[73] Rodriguez C, Mayo JC, Sainz RM, Antolin I, Herrera F, Martin V, et al. Regulation of antioxidant enzymes: a significant role for melatonin. Journal of Pineal Research. 2004;**36**:1-9. DOI: 10.1046/j.1600-079x.2003.00092.x

[74] Pieri C, Marra M, Moroni F, Recchioni R, Morcheselli F. Melatonin: a peroxyl radical scavenger more effective than vitamin E. Life Science. 1994;**55**: PL271-6. DOI: 10.1016/0024-3205(94)00666-0

[75] Reiter RJ, Manchester LC, Tan DX. Melatonin in walnuts: influence on levels of melatonin and total antioxidant capacity of blood. Nutrition. 2005;**21**:920-924. DOI: 10.1016/j.nut.2005.02.005

[76] Kumar A, Mehrotra S, Singh G, Mourya S, Narayanan K, Singh SK, Soni YK, Singh M, Mahla AS, Srivastava N, Verma MR. Sustained delivery of exogenous melatonin influences biomarkers of oxidative stress and total antioxidant capacity in summer stressed anoestrous water buffalo (*Bubalus bubalis*). Theriogenology. 2015;**83**:1402-1407. DOI: 10.1016/j.theriogenology.2014.12.023

[77] Ahmed WM, El-Khadrawy HH, El Hamed ABD, Amal R, Amer HA. Applied investigations on ovarian inactivity in buffalo heifers. International Journal of Academic Research. 2010;**2**:26

[78] Lucky HS, Gupta S, Kim Y, Agarwal A. Female infertility and antioxidants. Current Women's Health Reviews. 2010;**6**:84-95. DOI: 10.2174/157340410791321381

[79] Reynolds LP, Grazul-Bilska AT, Redmer DA. Angiogenesis in the female reproductive organs: pathological implications. International Journal of Experimental Pathology. 2002;**83**:151-164. DOI: 10.1046/j.1365-2613.2002.00277.x

[80] Rapoport R, Sklan D, Wolfenson D, Shaham-Albalancy A, Hanukoglu I. Antioxidant capacity is correlated with steroidogenic status of the corpus luteum during the bovine estrous cycle. Biochimica et Biophysica Acta. 1998;**1380**:133-140. DOI: 10.1016/s0304-4165(97)00136-0

[81] Sugino N, Takiguchi S, Kashida S, Karube A, Nakamura Y, Kato H. Superoxide dismutase expression in the human corpus luteum during the menstrual cycle and in early pregnancy. Molecular Human Reproduction. 2000;**6**:19-25. DOI: 10.1093/molehr/6.1.19

[82] Laloraya M, Kumar PG, Laloraya MM. Changes in the levels of superoxide anion radical and superoxide dismutase during the estrous cycle of Rattus norvegicus and induction of superoxide dismutase in rat ovary by lutropin. Biochemical and Biophysical Research Communications. 1988;**157**:146-153. DOI: 10.1016/s0006-291x(88)80025-1

[83] Singh J, Ghuman SPS, Cheema RS, Bansal AK. Melatonin implant induces estrus and alleviates oxidative stress in summer anestrus buffalo. Indian Journal of Animal Reproduction. 2016;**37**(2):28-32.

[84] Leon J, Acuna-Castroviejo D, Escames G, Tan DX, Reiter RJ. Melatonin mitigates mitochondrial malfunction. Journal of Pineal Research. 2005;**38**:1-9. DOI: 10.1111/j.1600-079x.2004.00181.x

[85] Rensis FD, Scaramuzzi RJ. Heat stress and seasonal effects on reproduction in the dairy cow—A review. Theriogenology. 2003;**60**:1139-1151. DOI: 10.1016/s0093-691x(03)00126-2

[86] Gimeno N, Landa A, Sterin-Speziale N, Cardinali D, Gimeno A. Melatonin blocks in vitro generation of prostaglandin by the uterus and hypothalamus. European Journal of Pharmacology. 1980;**62**:309-317. DOI:10.1016/0014-2999(80)90098-9

[87] Bojanowska E, Forsling M. The effects of melatonin on vasopressin secretion in vivo: interactions with acetylcholine and prostaglandins. Brain Research Bulletin. 1997;**42**:457-461. DOI: 10.1016/s0361-9230(96)00372-3

Chapter 6

Immunocastration as Alternative to Surgical Castration in Pigs

Marjeta Čandek-Potokar, Martin Škrlep and
Galia Zamaratskaia

Additional information is available at the end of the chapter

http://dx.doi.org/10.5772/intechopen.68650

Abstract

Surgical castration of piglets is a routine practice in pig production used to prevent the incidence of boar taint of pig meat, which may develop in entire male pigs as they reach puberty. This practice is being presently questioned in the European Union, and there is a strong initiative to end it. The initiative is presently voluntary; however, key stakeholders of European pig production sector have signed a declaration, and the actions undertaken by them already affect the business. Before such new concepts in pig production can be implemented, alternative solutions are needed, one of them being immunocastration. The present chapter will thus focus on the presentation of immunocastration as one of the promising alternatives to surgical castration. Theoretical and practical aspects of immunocastration in pig production will be described, and the advantages and disadvantages of this alternative will be summarised. Physiological principles of immunocastration and impacts on metabolism, growth performance, body composition and meat quality will be described and aspects of public acceptability reviewed.

Keywords: immunocastration, productivity, welfare, meat quality, public acceptance, pigs

1. Introduction

Castration of male piglets is a traditional practice in pig production used worldwide with the main goal to prevent boar taint of pig meat—an unpleasant odour refused by the majority of consumers [1]. Odour is an important sensory attribute that determines whether consumers will be satisfied with a meat product. In pork, odour can be adversely affected by accumulation of high levels of androstenone and/or skatole, the so-called boar taint [2, 3]. Androstenone is a testicular steroid (with no anabolic effects) and is described as having urine or sweat-like odour. It is produced by testicular Leydig cells of sexually mature males. Due to its lipophilic character, it accumulates in adipose tissue in much higher concentrations than other steroid hormones [4]. Androstenone is also secreted through saliva and serves as a pheromone to promote sexual behaviour in sows. On the other hand, skatole is produced in the intestine; its odour is related mostly to manure or, to a lesser extent, to naphthalene. Skatole has no known physiological function; it is toxic for most animals, but pigs are relatively resistant to it. It is a product of bacterial degradation of the amino acid tryptophan in the large intestine and is partly excreted through faeces, while the rest is absorbed in the blood and metabolised in the liver. Its hepatic metabolism is inhibited by steroid hormones (including androstenone). As a result, the increased concentrations of androstenone are responsible for higher levels of skatole [5]. Likewise skatole, due to its lipophilic nature, accumulates in the adipose tissue. The fat levels above which the consumers can detect the off-odour were determined to be in the range from 0.5 to 1.0 ppm for androstenone and in the range 0.2–0.25 ppm for skatole [6]. The major aspect determining the level of boar taint in pork is the balance between the biosynthesis and catabolism of androstenone and skatole. This balance is affected by various intrinsic and extrinsic factors (**Figure 1**) influenced mainly by pig genotype and nutrition (for review, see Refs. [5, 7]). Until recently, a traditional way to regulate boar taint was to modify gender by surgical castration of male pigs. Surgical castration prevents the formation of both androstenone and skatole; however, it is associated with productivity drawback, as it ceases the synthesis of testicular steroids including testosterone and oestrogens and therefore negatively affects lean tissue growth and feed efficiency. According to the legislation of the European Union (EU), surgical castration can be performed without the use of analgesia/anaesthesia within the first week after the birth of piglets [8]. Due to the pain induced during the procedure, there is a growing public criticism of this practice from pig welfare point of view [9, 10]. Thus, both economic and ethical concerns make it relevant to reconsider the need for surgical castration. As a consequence, a voluntary initiative has been launched by key stakeholders to stop castrating male piglets in the EU until 2018 [11]. However, to be able to stop castration, alternative methods are required to minimise the risk of boar taint. Ideally, these methods should be animal friendly, economically efficient and leading to production of high-quality

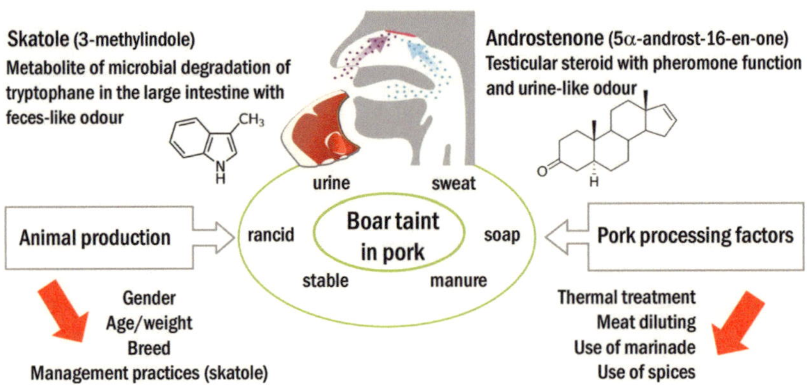

Figure 1. Boar taint: descriptors, responsible substances and influential factors.

and nutritious products. Among existing alternatives to surgical castration (**Table 1**), the so-called immunocastration, an active immunisation against gonadotropin-releasing hormone

Alternative		Advantage	Disadvantage
Castration	Surgical castration with anaesthesia and/or analgesia	Reduced pain during surgical castration	Increased costs, need for authorisation (drugs) and specially trained personnel
	Immunocastration	No castration pain and wounds Applicable for males and females Economic advantage of better performance Applicable for production systems with prolonged fattening	Need for authorisation (drugs) Need for safety measures for operators (self-injection) Questionable acceptability for consumers (and consequently chain actors)
Raising entire male pigs	Slaughter at younger age/lower weight (before puberty)	No conflict with animal welfare Reduced risk of high androstenone and skatole levels Economic advantage of better performance	No guarantee of total elimination of boar taint Lower technological meat quality Questionable economic efficiency
	Dietary manipulations	No conflict with animal welfare Reduced risk of high skatole levels Economic advantage of better performance	No guarantee of total elimination of boar taint Lower technological meat quality High costs of specific ingredients Not a solution for production systems with prolonged fattening
	Selection against boar taint	No conflict with animal welfare Reduced risk of high androstenone and skatole levels Economic advantage of better performance	No guarantee of total elimination of boar taint Lower technological meat quality Not a solution for production systems with prolonged fattening Reduced levels of anabolic hormones and, therefore, negative effects on growth performance of entire male pigs and onset of puberty in male and female pigs
Sex sorting	Sperm sexing	Production of female-only herds	High costs, low sperm output Technique for gender selection is not commercially available

Table 1. Cost-benefit analysis of available alternatives as compared to standard surgical castration of entire male piglets.

(GnRH; also referred to as gonadoliberin), is considered as an appropriate and one of the most attractive alternatives. Immunocastration hinders sex steroid synthesis, including androstenone production, along with a reduction of the size of reproductive organs, sperm number and aggressive behaviour [12–17]. Skatole levels are also reduced by immunocastration [13, 17–19]. The principle of immunocastration is based on the immunological blocking of the signal from GnRH, thus decreasing the secretion of luteinising hormone (LH) and follicle-stimulating hormone (FSH) and testicular steroids.

2. Reproductive physiology of boar

Puberty can be defined as series of physiological changes leading to full sexual maturity and capability of reproduction. It is accompanied by changes in testes structure and increased secretion of androgens and oestrogens. Puberty is heralded by an increase in the secretion of luteinising hormone (LH) and follicle-stimulating hormone (FSH) by the anterior pituitary gland. These processes are controlled by the extent and frequency of GnRH pulses, along with the feedback from androgens and estrogens. LH and FSH are responsible for the regulation of testicular function. The binding of LH to the receptors on the surface of the Leydig cells results in the induction of steroidogenic enzymes and increased levels of testicular steroids including androstenone. FSH affects the functioning of testicular Sertoli cells and is critical for the initiation of spermatogenesis. LH secretion is also controlled by some other hormones such as dopamine and prolactin and most crucially by negative feedback from sex steroids. It has also been shown that Leydig and Sertoli cells have receptors for growth factors including IGF-I [20]. In boars, growth hormone also stimulates functional maturation of Sertoli cells although without an effect on their number [21]. Thyroid hormones are also critically important for normal testicular development (of Sertoli cells and testes as a whole) [22]. Age-related variations of androstenone and testicular hormones are due to the common regulatory system controlling the biosynthesis of all testicular steroids. The synthesis of androstenone is low in young pigs (the transient increase in androstenone levels also occurs at the age of approximately 2–4 weeks due to Leydig cell activity at that time) but gradually increases simultaneously with other testicular steroids at puberty onset [23]. Therefore, puberty is a central stage of development regulating androstenone levels in entire male pigs by the maintenance of adult Leydig cell morphology and the stimulation of neuroendocrine system leading to increased biosynthesis of testicular steroids (mature boars show an increase in average Leydig cell size and therefore an increase in steroidogenic capacity per Leydig cell). In sexually mature boars, androstenone levels depend on the individual ability to produce this steroid.

In entire male pigs, androstenone is produced by the Leydig cells of the testes in parallel with anabolic testicular hormones [24]. Androstenone is synthesised from the precursors, pregnenolone and progesterone, through the formation of androstadienone by the sequential action of a number of enzymes, particularly cytochrome P450C17 and cytochrome b5 [25, 26]. Androstenone is metabolised in the liver with the production of alpha-androstenol and to a greater extent beta-androstenol [27, 28]. Part of androstenone is transported to the submaxillary salivary gland, where it is bind to a specific binding protein pheromaxein and released in

http://dx.doi.org/10.5772/intechopen.68650

the saliva, which among other 16-androstene steroids act as a pheromone to promote sexual behaviour in female pigs.

Hormonal regulation of boar taint is illustrated in **Figure 2**, which shows how androstenone biosynthesis is controlled through the activation of the hypothalamic-pituitary-gonadal axis. The level of skatole, the other boar taint compound, is also related to sexual maturation. Its accumulation in the adipose tissue is due to the inhibition of skatole metabolism in the liver by increased levels of testicular steroids, mainly androstenone [29] and oestrogens [30, 31], and in part also due to the effect of steroid hormones and growth factors on the epithelial proliferation and apoptosis in the intestine, the site of skatole formation [5].

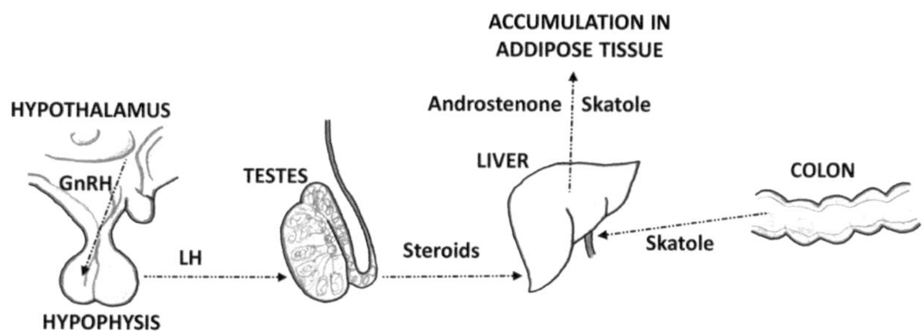

Figure 2. Relationships between the hypothalamic-pituitary-gonadal axis, androstenone production in testes and skatole formation from tryptophan in the intestine and their interrelated metabolism in the liver. In boar, the production of testicular steroids, including androstenone, inhibits hepatic clearance of skatole. Androstenone and skatole are accumulated in the adipose tissue due to their lipophilic nature.

3. Principles and effects of immunocastration

Immunocastration involves the vaccination of animals against hormones that control the reproductive function (**Figure 3**). Progress has lately been made to develop a vaccine for the immunisation against gonadotrophin-releasing hormone (GnRH). Commercially available vaccine (named Improvac in Europe, Improvest in the USA) against boar taint was developed in Australia and is now produced by Zoetis (formerly Pfizer Ltd., formerly CSL Limited, Parkville, Victoria, Australia). This vaccine was approved for use in pigs in many countries (including the EU from 2009), but its practical application is still limited.

Immunocastration uses the natural immune system of the animal to achieve the effects of castration. The vaccine contains physiologically inactive analogue of GnRH covalently conjugated to an immunogenic carrier protein. The analogue has no hormonal activity but contains the necessary epitopes to stimulate an effective anti-GnRH antibody response and blocks the stimulation of the hypothalamic-pituitary-gonadal axis. Consequently, the formation of gonadal steroid hormones is hindered and thereby the regression of reproductive organs and some induced metabolic changes, which ultimately leads to changes in behaviour (reduced aggression, increased appetite and feed intake) and growth performance [32].

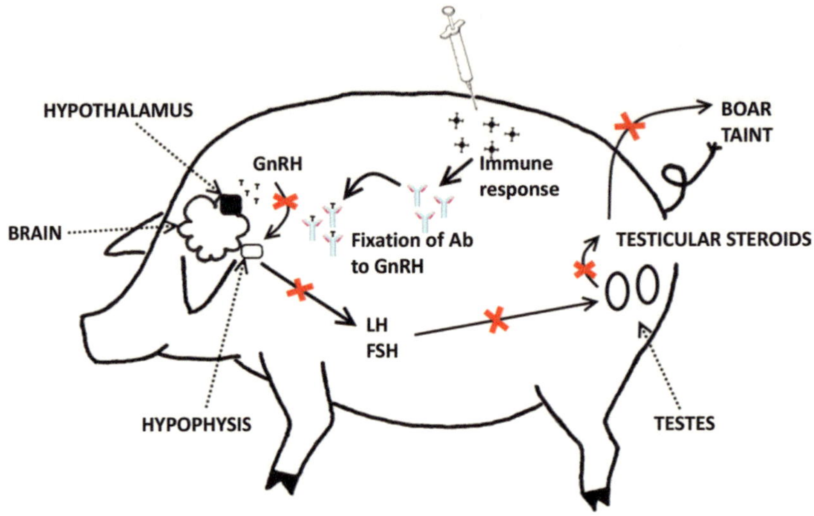

Figure 3. Physiological response to immunocastration in male pigs. The vaccine consists of the antigen (GnRH analogue that is bind to carrier protein), which triggers the immune system to produce antibodies that neutralise endogenous GnRH. Consequently, there is no stimulus for the hypophysis to release LH and FSH hormones, which in turn fails to signal the testes to produce testosterone and androstenone and thus prevents boar taint development.

3.1. Vaccination scheme

To achieve the effective immunisation, at least two applications of the vaccine with a minimum interval of 4 weeks are needed. Subcutaneous injections are given at the base of the ear with a special vaccinator designed by the vaccine producer to prevent accidental self-injection. The first dose primes the pig's immune system and can be given at any time after 8–9 weeks of age, and the second dose should be given (if we refer to standard pig production system where pigs are slaughtered at 6 months of age) no later than 4–5 weeks prior to slaughter. As the first injection has no apparent impact on steroid hormones, this schedule enables to use full growth potential of the entire male pigs until the second injection. After the immunisation, immunocastrated pigs rapidly change their metabolism to castrate-like, with increased feed consumption and fat deposition. The longer is the time elapsed from the second vaccination to slaughter, the higher is the difference between immunocastrates and entire males and/or the similarity to surgical castrates [33, 34]. In the case of older animals, a three-dose vaccination regimen might be required [35, 36] to ensure inactivation of endogenous GnRH and elimination of boar taint. Also, if nonrespondent pigs are detected (shown as larger testicle size or prolonged sexual behaviour), an additional dose might be applied [37].

A number of studies have been conducted using alternative vaccination schemes. A study conducted by Brunius et al. [38] investigated the efficacy of early vaccination with Improvac applied to entire male pigs at 10 and 14 weeks of age (pre- or early pubertal). It was shown that the levels of androstenone and skatole in pigs vaccinated at weeks 10 and 14 did not differ from the pigs vaccinated according to manufacturer's instructions. It has also been shown that already 2 weeks following the second vaccination, the levels of androstenone and skatole were below sensory threshold [33, 39]. The effect of immunocastration can last up to 22 weeks following the second injection [19].

3.2. Effect of immunocastration on boar taint compounds

Immunocastration blocks the synthesis of testicular steroids, including androstenone, by interfering with the hypothalamic-pituitary-gonadal axis. Androstenone production is suppressed as a consequence of suppressed testicular function. The approach with immunocastration therefore does not only prevent androstenone formation selectively but also reduces the synthesis of anabolic steroids.

Immunocastration also reduces the level of the another boar taint compound, skatole [13, 17, 18, 40]. Even though skatole is produced in the intestine by microbial degradation of amino acid tryptophan and the immunocastration has no direct effect on skatole synthesis, reduction of skatole levels in immunocastrated pigs is related to hindered production of androstenone and oestrogens. Androstenone and 17-beta-oestradiol were identified as potential inhibitors of the expression and/or activity of major skatole-metabolising enzymes CYP2E1 [29, 30, 41] and CYP2A [42]. Indeed, activities of skatole-metabolising enzymes in the liver are higher in surgically and immunocastrated male pigs than the entire male pigs [43, 44]. Thus, in the absence of androstenone and 17-beta-oestradiol, the hepatic metabolism of skatole is not inhibited, and produced skatole metabolites are readily eliminated from the body.

Generally, for what regards the prevention of boar taint in pork, immunocastration is comparable to surgical castration as similar effects are achieved as in physical removing of the testes.

3.3. Effect of immunocastration on growth performance and carcass quality

Considering the entire fattening period (from the first vaccination until slaughter), meta-analysis of the effects of immunocastration on pigs' growth showed that immunocastrates grow faster than surgical castrates and entire males [45]. The explanation is that immunocastrates are physiologically entire males until the second (effective) vaccination, and therefore until then, they exploit boar-like growth potential. Following the second vaccination, rapid changes of the hormonal status start, characterised by the drop of the steroid levels [46]. Simultaneously, the concentrations of residual IGF-1 and somatotropin remain relatively high [47, 48], resulting in higher feed intake and growth rate of immunocastrates after the effective immunisation is reached. A study of Batorek et al. [49] revealed that, after effective immunisation, the immunocastrates increase fat tissue deposition at the expense of lower heat production, while protein deposition remains similar to entire males and different from surgical castrates, which deposit fat instead of protein (i.e. muscles). It is, however, important to take into consideration that these results were obtained with late immunocastration, where the first vaccination is performed at the start of the fattening period and the second vaccination very late, usually 4–6 weeks prior to slaughter (i.e. may not be the case for early immunisation). Studies dealing with early immunocastration are rare as such practice is not economically interesting. The level of fat deposition in immunocastrates has been related to the delay between the second vaccination and slaughter; and with longer delay, higher fat deposition is reported [33, 34, 50]. Although intramuscular fat deposits are regarded as favourable for meat sensory quality, the overall increase in body adiposity has negative impacts on economics of rearing (higher fatness leads to lower lean meat %, governing the carcass price). Summarising 30 studies, the meta-analysis of Batorek et al. [45] showed that immunocastrates exhibit thicker back fat than entire males, resulting in lower carcass lean meat percentage. On the other hand, a comparison of immunocastrates with surgical castrates shows their advantages in terms of carcass quality (lower carcass fatness, heavier ham and shoulder). The way to control fat deposition in immunocastrates would be the manipulation of their diet after the second vaccination. Restricted feed intake [48] or energy dilution [51] improves carcass leanness due to lower fat deposition.

3.4. Effect of immunocastration on meat quality

Meta-analytical results [45, 52] show that immunocastrates and surgical castrates are very similar in regard to meat quality traits. On the other hand, compared to entire males (in addition to avoiding boar taint problem), immunocastrates exhibit superior meat quality as they have more intramuscular fat and more tender meat. Their fat is also more saturated, which is beneficial from the technological viewpoint. Besides that, unlike entire males, immunocastrates can be slaughtered at older age making their meat suitable for processing into dry-cured meat products, where raw material of specific quality is required. The available studies evaluating immunocastrates for dry-cured products show their similarity with surgical castrates in regard to meat and fat quality (including quantity and fatty acid composition) and are considered suitable for prolonged maturation process [36, 53–55]. A comparison of dry-cured hams originating from immunocastrates and entire males slaughtered at 130 kg [55] showed better aptitude of immunocastrates than entire males for long dry-curing maturation due to lower seasoning losses, lower salt intake and softer product with more intramuscular fat. However, it should be noted that fast changes of metabolism after the effective immunisation could reflect in changed protein turnover and consequently proteolytic activity of meat from immunocastrates, which is of relevance for long dry-curing process and would merit to be investigated for potential impact on product quality.

Due to the possible restauration of reproductive function and thus boar taint, triple vaccination protocol is considered in older, heavier pigs. Recent study comparing surgical castrates with double or triple vaccination [36] showed higher levels of boar taint compounds vaccinated only twice and slaughtered 14 weeks after the effective immunisation and concluded that three-dose immunocastration should be applied to meet the requirements for Italian PDO hams. The same study pointed out some indications of higher cathepsin activity than surgical castrates but only for immunocastrates vaccinated two times [36]. Similarly in the Iberian pigs [56, 57], the immunocastration with triple vaccination protocol has been found to be a suitable alternative as no major differences on carcass or technological and sensory meat quality were observed compared to surgically castrated females, whereas immunocastration of male pigs resulted in somewhat leaner carcasses with less intramuscular fat and lower tenderness than in surgical castrates.

Based on the studies, it can be concluded that the resemblance between immunocastrates and surgical castrates increases with the increase in elapsed time between the effective immunisation and slaughter. Depending on the need of pork industry, the protocol of vaccination can be adjusted (late or early vaccination, respectively). In summary, using immunocastration overcomes the drawbacks of pork production with entire males and is interesting for production systems with prolonged fattening (i.e. slaughter at higher age and weight) and extensive rearing systems.

3.5. Effect of immunocastration on animal welfare

Immunocastration itself, as a procedure, is considered a relatively welfare-friendly alternative. Compared to surgical castration without anaesthesia, it excludes acute pain associated with the procedure, the pain limited only to the needle insertion during application of the vaccine [10]. However, the administration in group-housing systems (or outdoor systems) may cause some practical difficulties that could trigger acute stress situations for pigs. The injection of the vaccine can also cause adverse reactions at the injection site, though these are most often reported as mild reactions [13, 58]. The injection of the vaccine is a systemic event leading to disturbance in the hormonal homeostasis of the animal; thus adverse effects could be expected in other tissues apart from the testes. One previous study suggested that immunisation against GnRH created tissue damages to the hypothalamus [59]. However, this was not confirmed in the later studies [60] likely due to improved vaccine formulation. The use of immunocastration on the other hand could overcome the mortality associated with surgical castration due to post-operation complications.

Until after the second administration of the vaccine, the immunocastrates are physiologically entire males, so compared to surgical castrates, they show male-like behaviour. This means more aggressive and mounting behaviour and higher number of skin lesions [61, 62]. However, after the second vaccination, aggressive and mounting behaviour is reduced to the level of surgically castrated pigs [63] in which standard production system happens in the period when aggressive behaviour would normally be intensified (i.e. at the age of 5–6 months). Soon after the effective immunisation, aggressive and mounting behaviour is reduced, while feeding behaviour becomes alike to surgical castrates [14, 19, 62]. Calmer behaviour is important for carcass quality because it is related to lower incidence of skin lesions, a consequence of fighting and mounting especially if unfamiliar pigs are mixed prior to slaughter (e.g. transport and lairage). Another aspect worth considering for the welfare of immunocastrates is related to their feeding. As their appetite is increased after the second vaccination, their feeding needs to be adapted to assure they are calm and satiety without negative effects on their body composition (energy dilution). Namely, restrictive feeding of immunocastrates showed similar level of aggression (i.e. incidence of carcass skin lesions) in restrictively fed immunocastrates as in entire males and higher as in ad libitum fed immunocastrates and surgical castrates [48].

4. Immunocastration and public acceptability

Despite the fact that the vaccine for immunocastration has been available in the European Union since 2009, its practical use is limited due to a generally low market acceptance [64]. Surveys with European stakeholders performed within PIGCAS project showed low prospects for immunocastration (surgical castration with anaesthesia/analgesia was preferred). It is also indicated that the main drawback of the immunocastration was the fear of consumers' acceptance [65]. However, opinion of consumers about immunocastration has not been thoroughly investigated, and they are mostly not well informed about boar taint and the methods used to prevent it [32, 66]. Consumers expect healthy, safe and tasty meat, which denotes that boar taint represents an important concern for consumer acceptance [32]. Presently available studies about the consumer acceptability of the immunocastration show important differences across Europe. For Swiss consumers, the most acceptable alternative was surgical castration with anaesthesia/analgesia, while immunocastration was not favoured [67]. Swedish consumers expressed preference for meat from immunocastrates over the entire males and standard surgical castrates [68]. Belgian consumers, after being well informed on the existing alternatives, preferred immunocastration to surgical castration [69]. The same was observed for German consumers [70]. A survey with over 4000 consumers in France, Germany and the Netherlands [71] pointed out that the fear of negative consumer attitude towards immunocastration might be overestimated. Namely, in this survey immunocastration was acceptable for over 70% of the respondents. It is worth noting that a recent study [64] reported that Belgian farmers changed their attitude after having used different alternatives in a real life scenario and preferred entire males and immunocastration. For them, surgical castration with anaesthesia and/or analgesia was the least acceptable due to being the most demanding (labour intensive, costly and complex). In Belgium, immunocastration is practised by some farmers since 2011 because of retailers' demand [64]. Regarding other stakeholders, nongovernmental animal welfare organisations find immunocastration acceptable, although they prioritise rearing of entire males. According to PIGCAS project survey, the scientists perceive immunocastration as a better alternative to surgical castration with anaesthesia/analgesia due to being more practical and having benefits for animal welfare and economics [72]. Overall, it seems that the main obstacle for wider utilisation of the immunocastration resides in the fear of consumers and how they would accept this alternative. Other drawbacks expressed by stakeholders are related to the ease of use in group-housing or outdoor production systems and security at work (fear of self-vaccination).

5. Tools to assess effectiveness of immunocastration

Several studies have shown that the effect of immunocastration is very consistent among individuals. However, there are cases where nonresponders (0–3%) have been reported [39, 54, 73] in both small- and large-scale experiments. The reasons why some pigs escape the vaccination have not yet been sufficiently explained but may be ascribed to poor health status or malnutrition of the pig or the fact that some pigs are simply missed at physical vaccination in group-housing systems. This argues for the development of good tools to assess the effectiveness of immunocastration, e.g. at the slaughter line. Assessing the effectiveness of vaccination in live pigs basing on the observation of testes size or taking blood for hormonal analyses is practically difficult and economically unsustainable. Behavioural observations like high rates of mounting could also be warning signs used at the farm to detect possible nonresponders; however, this later is not very practical in large-scale farming systems. After the slaughter, a reliable method would be to chemically determine the level of boar taint compounds in fat tissue; however, for practical and economic reasons, simple, low-cost online methods are desired. One option would be to monitor the size and weight of the testes, which have been shown to decrease significantly with successful immunocastration. However, as size/weight of testes is strongly related to pig's weight, it may not be a sufficiently reliable indicator of successful vaccination because of partly overlapping distributions between successfully immunocastrated and entire male pigs [17]. It was suggested that measuring seminal vesicle weight at slaughter line is more reliable to identify nonresponders [74]. A recent study [75] showed 100% success rate for prediction of nonresponders by combining the information on weight of all reproductive organs. In addition to morphological assessment of the size of reproductive organs at slaughter line, suspicious carcasses of immunocastrates could be additionally checked for boar taint by rapid methods involving the heating of fat tissue and sniffing.

Acknowledgements

This work is dedicated to the memory of Professor Kerstin Lundström. During the work at Swedish University of Agricultural Sciences, Professor Kerstin Lundström made a significant contribution to the many fields of meat science. Particularly, Prof. Lundström had an extremely high international reputation as a researcher on boar taint and friendly alternatives to surgical castration of entire male pigs, including immunocastration. Prof. Lundström will be remembered as a committed researcher and an outstanding specialist.

The support of COST action CA15215 Innovative approaches in pork production with entire males (IPEMA) is greatly acknowledged. M. Čandek-Potokar and M. Škrlep received financial support from Slovenian Agency of Research (core-financing grant P4-0133, project grant L4-5521) and Ministry of Agriculture, Food and Forestry. G. Zamaratskaia would like to acknowledge the financial support of the Ministry of Education, Youth and Sports of the Czech Republic via Projects "CENAKVA" (No. CZ.1.05/2.1.00/01.0024) and "CENAKVA II" (No. LO1205 under the NPU I program).

Author details

Marjeta Čandek-Potokar[1,2]*, Martin Škrlep[1] and Galia Zamaratskaia[3,4]

*Address all correspondence to: meta.candek-potokar@kis.si

1 Agricultural Institute of Slovenia, Ljubljana, Slovenia

2 Faculty of Agriculture and Life Sciences, University of Maribor, Hoče, Slovenia

3 Swedish University of Agricultural Sciences, Department of Molecular Sciences, Uppsala, Sweden

4 Faculty of Fisheries and Protection of Waters, South Bohemian Research Center of Aquaculture and Biodiversity of Hydrocenoses, University of South Bohemia in České Budějovice, Vodnany, Czech Republic

References

[1] Weiler U, Font i Furnols M, Fischer K, Kemmer H, Oliver MA, Gispert M. Influence of differences in sensitivity of Spanish and German consumers to perceive androstenone on the acceptance of boar meat differing in skatole and androstenone concentrations. Meat Science. 2000;**54**:297-304. DOI: 10.1016/S0309-1740(99)00106-0

[2] Patterson RLS. 5α-androst-16-ene-3-one: Compound responsible for taint in boar fat. Journal of Science of Food and Agriculture. 1968;**19**:31-38. DOI: 10.1002/jsfa.2740190107

[3] Walstra P, Maarse G. Onderzoek gestachlengen van mannelijke mestvarkens. Researchgroep voor Vlees en Vleeswaren TNO, IVO-rapport C-147, 1970. Rapport 2. p. 30

[4] Gower DB. 16-Unsaturated C 19 steroids. A review of their chemistry, biochemistry and possible physiological role. Journal of Steroid Biochemistry. 1972;**3**:45-103. DOI: 10.1016/0022-4731(72)90011-8

[5] Zamaratskaia G, Squires EJ. Biochemical, nutritional and genetic effects on boar taint in entire male pigs. Animal. 2009;**3**:1508-1521. DOI: 10.1017/S1751731108003674

[6] Walstra P, Claudi-Magnussen C, Chevillon P, von Seth G, Diestre A, Matthews KR, Homer DB, Bonneau M. An international study on the importance of androstenone and skatole for boar taint: Levels of androstenone and skatole by country and season. Livestock Production Science. 1999;**62**:15-28. DOI: 10.1016/S0301-6226(99)00054-8

[7] Wesoly R, Weiler U. Nutritional influences on skatole formation and skatole metabolism in the pig. Animal. 2012;**2**:221-242. DOI: 10.3390/ani2020221

[8] Council Directive 2008/120/EC of 18 December 2008 laying down minimum standards for the protection of pigs. Official Journal of the European Union. 2009;**52**:5-13

[9] McGlone JJ, Nicholson RI, Hellman JM, Herzog DN. The development of pain in young pigs associated with castration and attempts to prevent castration-induced behavioral changes. Journal of Animal Science. 1993;**71**:1441-1446. DOI: 10.2527/1993.7161441x

[10] Prunier A, Bonneau M, von Borell EH, Cinotti S, Gunn M, Fredriksen B, Giershing M, Morton DB, Tuyttens FAM, Velarde A. A review of the welfare consequences of surgical castration in piglets and the evaluation of non-surgical methods. Animal Welfare. 2006;**15**:277-289

[11] European Declaration on Alternatives to Surgical Castration of Pigs. 2010. Available from: http://ec.europa.eu/food/animals/welfare/practice/farm/pigs/castration_alternatives_en [Accessed: 18-01-2017]

[12] Bonneau M, Dufour R, Chouvet C, Roulet C, Meadus W, Squires EJ. The effects of immunization against luteinizing hormone-releasing hormone on performance, sexual development, and levels of boar taint-related compounds in intact male pigs. Journal of Animal Science. 1994;**72**:14-20. DOI: 10.2527/1994.72114x

[13] Dunshea FR, Colantoni C, Howard K, McCauley I, Jackson P, Long KA, Lopaticki S, Nugent EA, Simons JA, Walker J, Hennessy DP. Vaccination of boars with a GnRH vaccine (Improvac) eliminates boar taint and increases growth performance. Journal of Animal Science. 2001;**79**:2524-2535. DOI: 10.2527/2001.79102524x

[14] Cronin GM, Dunshea FR, Butler KL, McCauly I, Branett JL, Hemsworth PH. The effects of immuno- and surgical castration on the behaviour and consequently growth of group-housed, male finisher pigs. Applied Animal Behaviour Science. 2003;**81**:111-126. DOI: 10.1016/S0168-1591(02)00256-3

[15] Oliver WT, McCauley I, Harrell RJ, Suster D, Kerton DJ, Dunshea FR. A gonadotropin-releasing factor vaccine (Improvac) and porcine somatotropin have synergistic and additive effects on growth performance in group-housed boars and gilts. Journal of Animal Science. 2003;**81**:1959-1966. DOI: 10.2527/2003.8181959x

[16] Jaros P, Bürgi E, Stärk KDC, Claus R, Hennessy D, Thun R. Effect of active immunization against GnRH on androstenone concentration, growth performance and carcass quality in intact male pigs. Livestock Production Science. 2005;**92**:31-38. DOI: 10.1016/j.livprodsci.2004.07.011

[17] Zamaratskaia G, Andersson HK, Chen G, Andersson K, Madej A, Lundström K. Effect of a gonadotropin-releasing hormone vaccine (Improvac®) on steroid hormones, boar taint and performance in entire male pigs. Reproduction in Domestic Animals. 2008;**43**:351-359. DOI: 10.1111/j.1439-0531.2007.00914.x

[18] Metz C, Hohl K, Waidelich S, Drochner W, Claus R. Active immunization of boars against GnRH at an early age: consequences for testicular function, boar taint accumulation and N-retention. Livestock Production Science. 2002;**74**:147-157. DOI: 10.1016/S0301-6226(01)00292-5

[19] Zamaratskaia G, Rydhmer L, Andersson HK, Chen G, Lowagie S, Andersson K, Lundström K. Long-term effect of vaccination against gonadotropin-releasing hormone, using Improvac TM, on hormonal profile and behaviour of male pigs. Animal Reproduction Science. 2008;**108**:37-48. DOI: 10.1016/j.anireprosci.2007.07.001

[20] Hafez ESE. Anatomy of male reproduction. In: Hafez B, Hafez ESE, editors. Reproduction in Farm Animals. 7th ed. Baltimore: Lippincott Williams and Wilkins; 2000. pp. 1-12

[21] Swanlund DJ, N'Diaye MR, Loseth KJ, Pryor JL, Crabo BG. Diverse testicular responses to exogenous growth hormone and follicle-stimulating hormone in prepubertal boars. Biology of Reproduction. 1995;**53**:749-757. DOI: 10.1095/biolreprod53.4.749

[22] Cooke PS. Thyroid hormone and the regulation of testicular development. Animal Reproduction Science. 1996;**42**:333-341. DOI: 10.1016/0378-4320(96)01489-3

[23] Claus R, Weiler U, Herzog A. Physiological aspects of androstenone and skatole formation in the boar-a review with experimental data. Meat Science. 1994;**38**:289-305. DOI: 10.1016/0309-1740(94)90118-X

[24] Kwan TK, Orengo C, Gower DB. Biosynthesis of androgens and pheromonal steroids in neonatal porcine testicular preparations. FEBS Letters. 1985;**183**:359-364. DOI: 10.1016/0014-5793(85)80810-3

[25] Meadus WJ, Mason JI, Squires EJ. Cytochrome P450c17 from porcine and bovine adrenal catalyses the formation of 5,16 androstadien-3b-ol from pregnenolone in the presence of cytochrome b5. Journal of Steroid Biochemistry and Molecular Biology. 1993;**46**:565-572. DOI: 10.1016/0960-0760(93)90183-W

[26] Davis SM, Squires EJ. Association of cytochrome b5 with 16- androstene steroid synthesis in the testis and accumulation in the fat of male pigs. Journal of Animal Science. 1999;**77**:1230-1235. DOI: 10.2527/1999.7751230x

[27] Bonneau M, Terqui MA. A note on the metabolism of 5-androst-16-en-3-one in the young boar in vivo. Reproduction Nutrition Development. 1983;**23**:899-905. DOI: 10.1051/rnd: 19830610

[28] Doran E, Whittington FM, Wood JD, McGivan JD. Characterization of androstenone metabolism in pig liver microsomes. Chemico-Biological Interactions. 2004;**147**:141-149. DOI: 10.1016/j.cbi.2003.12.002

[29] Tambyrajah WS, Doran E, Wood JD, McGivan JD. The pig CYP2E1 promoter is activated by COUP-TF1 and HNF-1 and is inhibited by androstenone. Archives of Biochemistry and Biophysics. 2004;**431**:252-260. DOI: 10.1016/j.abb.2004.08.016

[30] Zamaratskaia G, Gilmore WJ, Lundström K, Squires EJ. Effect of testicular steroids on catalytic activities of cytochrome P450 enzymes in porcine liver microsomes. Food and Chemical Toxicology. 2007;**45**:676-681. DOI: 10.1016/j.fct.2006.10.023

[31] Rasmussen MK, Zamaratskaia G, Ekstrand B. In vitro cytochrome P450 2E1 and 2A activities in the presence of testicular steroids. Reproduction in Domestic Animals. 2011;**46**:149-154. DOI: 10.1111/j.1439-0531.2010.01613.x

[32] Škrlep M, Batorek Lukač N, Prevolnik Povše M, Čandek-Potokar M. Theoretical and practical aspects of immunocastration. Stočarstvo. 2014;**68**:39-49

[33] Lealiifano AK, Pluske JR, Nicholls RR, Dunshea FR, Campbell RG, Hennessy DP, Miller DW, Hansen CF, Mullan BP. Reducing the length of time between slaughter and the secondary gonadotropin-releasing factor immunization improves the growth performances and clears boar taint compounds in male finishing pigs. Journal of Animal Science. 2011;**89**:2782-2792. DOI: 10.2527/jas.2010-3267

[34] Škrlep M, Čandek-Potokar M, Batorek N, Šegula B, Prevolnik M, Pugliese C, Bonneau M. Length of the interval between immunocastration and slaughter in relation to boar taint and carcass traits. In: 20th International Symposium Animal Science Days; 19-21 September 2012; Kranjska Gora, Slovenia. Ljubljana: Biotechnical Faculty; 2012. Acta agriculturae Slovenica, suppl. 3. 247-251

[35] Allison J, Tolasi G, Solari Basano F, Nazzari R, Minelli G, Pearce M. Efficacy of Improvac for controlling boar taint in heavy male pigs under commercial field conditions in Italy. In: Proceedings of the 55th International Congress of Meat Science and Technology (ICoMST); 16-21 August 2009; Copenhagen, Denmark, PE1.09; 2009. pp. 64-67

[36] Pinna A, Schivazappa C, Virgili R, Parolari G. Effect of vaccination against gonadotropin-releasing hormone (GnRH) in heavy male pigs for Italian typical dry-cured ham production. Meat Science. 2015;**110**:153-169. DOI: doi.org/10.1016/j.meatsci.2015.07.002

[37] Hennessy D. Global control of boar taint. Part 4. Immunological castration in action. Pig Progress. 2006;**22**:14-16

[38] Brunius C, Zamaratskaia G, Andersson K, Chen G, Norrby M, Madej A, Lundström K. Early immunocastration of male pigs with Improvac - effect on boar taint, hormones and reproductive organs. Vaccine. 2011;**29**:9514-9520. DOI: 10.1016/j.vaccine.2011.10.014

[39] Kubale V, Batorek N, Škrlep M, Prunier A, Bonneau M, Fazarinc G, Čandek-Potokar M. Steroid hormones, boar taint compounds, and reproductive organs in pigs according to the delay between immunocastration and slaughter. Theriogenology. 2013;**79**:69-80. DOI: 10.1016/j.theriogenology.2012.09.010

[40] Hennessy DP, Colantoni C, Dunshea FR, Howard K, Jackson P, Long K, Lopaticki S, Sali L, Simons J, Walker J. Elimination of boar taint: A commercial boar taint vaccine for male pigs. In: Bonneau M, Lundström K, Malmfors B, editors. Boar Taint in Entire Male Pigs. No. 92. Wageningen: EAAP Publications; 1997. pp. 141-217

[41] Doran E, Whittington FW, Wood JD, McGivan JD. Cytochrome P450IIE1 (CYP2E1) is induced by skatole and this induction is blocked by androstenone in isolated pig hepatocytes. Chemico-Biological Interactions. 2002;**140**:81-92. DOI: 10.1016/S0009-2797(02)00015-7

[42] Chen G, Cue R-A, Lundström K, Wood JH, Doran O. Regulation of cytochrome P450 2A6 protein expression by skatole, indole and testicular steroids in primary cultured porcine hepatocytes. Drug Metabolism and Disposition. 2008;**36**:56-60. DOI: 10.1124/dmd.107.017285

[43] Zamaratskaia G, Zlabek V, Chen G, Madej A. Modulation of porcine cytochrome P450 enzyme activities by surgical castration and immunocastration. Animal. 2009;**3**:1124-1132. DOI: 10.1017/S1751731109004510

[44] Brunius C, Rasmussen MK, Ekstrand B, Lacoutiere H, Andersson K, Zamaratskaia G. Expression and activities of hepatic cytochrome P450 (CYP1A, CYP2A and CYP2E1) in entire and castrated male pigs. Animal. 2012;**6**:271-277. DOI:10.1017/S1751731111001674

[45] Batorek N, Čandek-Potokar M, Bonneau M, Van Milgen J. Meta-analysis of the effect of immunocastration on production performance, reproductive organs and boar taint compounds in pigs. Animal. 2012;**6**:1330-1338. DOI: 10.1017/S1751731112000146

[46] Claus R, Lacorn M, Danowski K, Pearce MC, Bauer A. Short-term endocrine and metabolic reactions before and after second immunisation against GnRH in boars. Vaccine. 2007;**25**:4689-4696. DOI: 10.1016/j.vaccine.2007.04.009

[47] Metz C, Claus R. Active immunization of boars against GnRH does not affect growth hormone but lowers IGF-I in plasma. Livestock Production Science. 2003;**81**:129-137. DOI: 10.1016/S0301-6226(02)00302-0

[48] Batorek N, Škrlep M, Prunier A, Louveau I, Noblet J, Bonneau M, Čandek-Potokar M. Effect of feed restriction on hormones, performance, carcass traits, and meat quality in immunocastrated pigs. Journal of Animal Science. 2012;**90**:4593-4603. DOI: 10.2527/jas2012-5330

[49] Batorek N, Noblet J, Dubois S, Bonneau M, Čandek-Potokar M, Labussiere E. Effect of immunocastration in combination with addition of fat to diet on quantitative oxidation of nutrients and fat retention in male pigs. In: Oltjen JW, Kebreab E, Lapierre H, editors. Energy and Protein Metabolism and Nutrition in Sustainable Animal Production. Vol. 134. Wageningen: Wageningen Academic Publishers; 2013. pp. 185-186. DOI: 10.3920/978-90-8686-781-3_55

[50] Turkstra JA, Zeng XY, Diepen JTM, van Jongbloed AW, Oonk HB, van de Viel DFM, Meloen RH. Performance of male pigs immunised against GnRH is related to time of the onset of biological response. Journal of Animal Science. 2002;**80**:2953-2959. DOI: 10.2527/2002.80112953x

[51] Batorek N, Noblet J, Bonneau M, Čandek-Potokar M, Labussiere E. Effect of dietary net energy content on performance and lipid deposition in immunocastrated pigs. In: Book of Abstracts of the 64th Annual Meeting of the European Federation of Animal Science; 26-30 August 2013; Nantes, France. Wageningen: Wageningen Academic Publishers; 2013. p. 560

[52] Trefan L, Doeschl-Wilson A, Rooke JA, Terlouw C, Bünger L. Meta-analysis of effects of gender in combination with carcass weight and breed on pork quality. Journal of Animal Science. 2013;**91**:1480-1492. DOI: 10.2527/jas.2012-5200

[53] Font-i-Furnols M, González J, Gispert M, Oliver MA, Hortós M, Pérez J, Guerrero L. Sensory characterization of meat from pigs vaccinated against gonadotropin releasing factor compared to meat from surgically castrated, entire male and female pigs. Meat Science. 2009;**83**:438-442. DOI: 10.1016/j.meatsci.2009.06.020

[54] Font-i-Furnols M, Gispert M, Soler J, Diaz M, Garcia-Regueiro JA, Diaz I, Pearce MC. Effect of vaccination against gonadotrophin-releasing factor on growth performance, carcass, meat and fat quality of male Duroc pigs for dry-cured ham production. Meat Science. 2012;**91**:148-154. DOI: 10.1016/j.meatsci.2012.01.008

[55] Škrlep M, Čandek-Potokar M, Batorek Lukač N, Prevolnik Povše M, Pugliese C, Labussiere E, Flores M. Comparison of entire male and immunocastrated pigs for dry-cured ham production under two salting regimes. Meat Science. 2016;**111**:27-36. DOI: 10.1016/j.meatsci.2015.08.010

[56] Martinez-Macipe M, Rodríguez P, Izquierdo M, Gispert M, Manteca X, Mainauc E, Hernández FI. Comparison of meat quality parameters in surgical castrated versus vaccinated against gonadotropin-releasing factor male and female Iberian pigs reared in free-ranging conditions. Meat Science. 2016;**111**:116-121. DOI: 10.1016/j.meatsci.2015.09.002

[57] Izquierdo M, Pérez MA, Del Rosario AI, Rodriguez P, García J, Duarte JL, Dalmau A, Hernández-García FI. The effect of immunocastration on carcass and meat cut yields in extensively reared Iberian gilts. In: 8th International Symposium on the Mediterranean Pig; 10-12 October 2013; Ljubljana, Slovenia. Ljubljana: Biotechnical Faculty; 2013. Acta Agriculturae Slovenica, suppl. 4. 205-209

[58] Einarsson S. Vaccination against GnRH: pros and cons. Acta Veterinaria Scandinavica. 2006;**48**(Suppl. 1):S10. DOI: 10.1186/1751-0147-48-S1-S10

[59] Molenaar GJ, Lugard-Kok C, Meloen RH, Oonk RB, de Koning J, Wessing CJG. Lesions in the hypothalamus after active immunisation against GnRH in the pig. Journal of Neuroimmunology. 1993;**48**:1-11. DOI: 10.1016/0165-5728(93)90052-Z

[60] Hilbe M, Jaros P, Ehrensperger F, Zlinszky K, Janett F, Hässig M, Thun R. Histomorphological and immunohistochemical findings in testes, bulbourethral glands and brain of immunologically castrated male piglets. Schweizer Archiv für Tierheilkunde. 2006;**148**:599-608. DOI: 10.1024/0036-7281.148.11.599

[61] Andersson K, Brunius C, Zamaratskaia G Lundström K. Early vaccination with Improvac®: Effects on performance and behaviour of male pigs. Animal. 2012;**6**:87-95. DOI: 10.1017/S1751731111001200

[62] Rydhmer L, Lundström K, Andersson K. Immunocastration reduces aggressive and sexual behaviour in male pigs. Animal. 2010;**4**:965-972. DOI: 10.1017/S175173111000011X

[63] Karaconji B, Lloyd B, Campbell N, Meaney D, Ahern T. Effect of an anti-gonadotropin-releasing factor vaccine on sexual and aggressive behaviour in male pigs during the finishing period under Australian field conditions. Australian Veterinary Journal. 2015;**93**: 121-123. DOI: 10.1111/avj.12307

[64] Aluwé M, Tuyttens FAM, Millet S. Field experience with surgical castration with anaesthesia, analgesia, immunocastration and production of entire male pigs: Performance, carcass traits and boar taint prevalence. Animal. 2015;**9**:500-508. DOI: 10.1017/S1751731114002894

[65] Bonneau M, Oliver MA, Fredriksen B, Edwards SA, Ouedraogo A, Spoolder H, von Borell E, Lundström K, de Roest K, Prunier A, Tuyttens FAM, Migdal W, Font i Furnols M. PIGCAS, Attitudes, Practices and State of the Art Regarding Piglet Castration in Europe. Report on Recommendations for Research and Policy Support. 2009. Available from: http://w3.rennes.inra.fr/pigcas/ [Accessed: 12-10-2013]

[66] Kallas Z, Gil JM, Panella-Riera N, Blanch M, Font-i-Furnols M, Chevillon P, De Roest K, Tacken G, Oliver MA. Effect of tasting and information on consumer opinion about pig castration. Meat Science. 2013;**95**:242-249. DOI: 10.1016/j.meatsci.2013.05.011

[67] Huber-Eicher B, Spring P. Attitudes of Swiss consumers towards meat from entire or immunocastrated boars: A representative survey. Research in Veterinary Science. 2008;**85**:625-627. DOI: 10.1016/j.rvsc.2008.03.002

[68] Lagerkvist CJ. Swedish consumer preferences for animal welfare and biotech: A choice experiment. AgBioForum. 2006;**9**:51-58

[69] Tuyttens FAM, Vanhonacker F, Langendries K, Aluwé M, Millet S, Bekaert K, Verbeke W. Effect of information provisioning on attitude toward surgical castration of male piglets and alternative strategies for avoiding boar taint. Research in Veterinary Science. 2011;**91**:327-332. DOI: 10.1016/j.rvsc.2011.01.005

[70] Sattler T, Schmoll F. Impfung oder Kastration zur Vermeidung von Ebergeruch – Ergebnisse einer repräsentativen Verbraucherumfrage in Deutschland. Journal für Verbraucherschutz und Lebensmittelsicherheit. 2012;**7**:117-123. DOI: 10.1007/s00003-012-0767-y

[71] Vanhonacker F, Verbeke W. Consumer response to the possible use of vaccine method to control boar taint v. Physical piglet castration with anaesthesia: A quantitative study in four European countries. Animal. 2011;**5**:1107-1118. DOI: 10.1017/S1751731111000139

[72] Edwards SA, Oliver MA, Ouedraogo A, Gonzalez J, Gil M, Fredriksen B, von Borell E, Baumgartner J, Giershing M, Jaeggin N, Prunier A, Tuyttens FAM, Spoolder H, Lundström K, Zamaratskaia G, Matthews K, Haugen JE, Squires EJ, de Roest K, Montanari C, Fowler T, Baltussen W, Migdal W, Font i Furnols M, Bonneau M. PIGCAS, Attitudes, Practices and State of the Art Regarding Piglet Castration in Europe. Report on Evaluation of Research and Other Information. 2009. Available from: http://w3.rennes.inra.fr/pigcas [Accessed: 12-10-2013]

[73] Škrlep M, Batorek N, Bonneau M, Prevolnik M, Kubale V, Čandek-Potokar M. Effect of immunocastration in group-housed commercial fattening pigs on reproductive organs, malodorous compounds, carcass and meat quality. Czech Journal of Animal Science. 2012;**57**:290-299

[74] Bonneau M. Accessory sex glands as a tool to measure the efficacy of immunocastration in male pigs. Animal. 2010;**4**:930-932. DOI: 10.1017/S1751731110000091

[75] Čandek-Potokar M, Prevolnik M, Škrlep M. Testes weight is not a reliable tool for discriminating immunocastrates from entire males. In: Proceedings of the International Symposium of Animal Science; 23-25 September 2014; Belgrade, Serbia. Belgrade: Faculty of Agriculture, 2014. pp. 43-49

Section 2

Topics from Aquatic Systems

Chapter 7

Ovary Differentiation and Activity in Teleostei Fish

Talita Sarah Mazzoni and Irani Quagio Grassiotto

Additional information is available at the end of the chapter

http://dx.doi.org/10.5772/intechopen.69022

Abstract

Teleostei fishes constitute a very large group among the vertebrates. They present several reproductive strategies, and many species are gonochoristics. During the gonadal differentiation, the gonadal primordium undergoes morphological changes giving rise to male or female gonads. Considering the lack of information about gonadal morphogenesis in Teleostei, especially in tangent aspects concerning the establishment of the germinal epithelium and its relation with the formation of the ovarian cavity, *Tanichthys albonubes*, *Corydoras schwartzi*, and *Amatitlania nigrofasciata* were taken as biological models to establish a comparative analysis of the female gonadal differentiation. In undifferentiated gonad, the epithelial cells associate with primordial germ cells and form germline cysts. These are distributed throughout the gonadal tissue; after the entrance of the oogonia into meiosis, the folliculogenesis occurs forming the first follicles, in a quite conserved process. However, the formation of the ovarian cavity is distinct. In *T. albonubes* and *A. nigrofasciata*, the lumen is formed by pleating and in *C. schwartzi*, it is formed by cavitation. The central lumen formed characterizes the cystovarian of Teleostei. Although there are differences in the chronology of the differentiation, the processes involved are quite similar and culminate in the formation of analogous structures.

Keywords: germinal epithelium, gonadal differentiation, germline cysts, folliculogenesis, cystovarian formation, Teleostei fish

1. Introduction

Teleostei fish represents about 50% of the vertebrates [1]. The bony fishes, within the Teleostei, are divided into Ostariophysi, Protacanthopterygii, and Neoteleostei.

Ostariophysi is the second largest superorder of fish, and it is considered the most basal among the Teleostei, representing about three quarters of the world's freshwater fish [1]. This diverse group contains important fish in the area of feeding, sport fishing, aquarium, and research, such as the common carp and zebrafish (Cypriniformes), the characids and tetras (Characiformes), the catfishes (Siluriformes), and the electric eels (Gymnotiformes) [1, 2].

The Neoteleostei is another large clade of bony fish that includes most derived species among Teleostei, and it is also very important in several areas. Among the Neoteleostei, the most relevant group is the Perciformes, which presents the greatest diversity among all orders of fish, being the largest order among vertebrates [1]. The most popular Perciformes are the cichlids, such as tilapia.

Regardless of their position on the phylogenetic scale, in most Teleostei species, the reproduction is cyclic and seasonal, determining a series of morphophysiological modifications in their gonads [3]. Teleostei present several reproductive strategies [3, 4]. Among these, there are mechanisms of release of gametes in the aquatic environment for external fertilization, development of specialized organs for internal fertilization, posture of fertilized eggs after internal fertilization, and even internal gestation of the embryos [5].

In Teleostei, the sexual determination and gonadal differentiation are controlled by genetic, physiological, and behavioral factors [6]. The genetic sex of the embryo is determined at the time of the fertilization by the combination of the chromosomes from the male and female gametes, and sexual determination is defined as the sum of the genes responsible for the formation of the gonads and their characteristics [7, 8]. In this aspect, the genetic control is one of the main determinants of the gender, even though environmental factors, such as temperature, photoperiod, or salinity, also have a great influence on the process, determining the physiological gender of the fish [9].

Most Teleostei are dioecious or gonochoristic, that is, they present individuals with separated sexes. These fishes may present two types of gonadal development, classified as undifferentiated or differentiated gonochoristics. In undifferentiated gonochoristics, the undifferentiated gonad begins its development resembling an ovary. Subsequently, part of the individuals becomes male, while another part remains female. This natural condition is known as juvenile hermaphroditism. In the differentiated gonochoristics, the gonad differentiates directly in a testis or in an ovary [6, 10].

However, at the beginning of embryogenesis, the gender of the fish is not morphologically defined, since it does not have gonads differentiated in testes or ovaries, and there is no other developed characteristic which is associated to the reproductive system. There are only embryological precursors that will give rise to the ovaries and testes: the primordial germ cells (PGCs) and the somatic cells. At this stage of development, these cells are totipotent, and they can give rise to male or female gonads [6]. At some point during gonadal development, through hormonal chemical signaling, the gonad differentiates into the ovary or testis. Once this occurs and the gonadal tissue completes its differentiation, the fish becomes physiologically male or female [11].

The gonadal differentiation in the Teleostei includes changes in both somatic and germ cells [9], as mitotic divisions of oogonia or spermatogonia from the primordial germ cells, to structural changes, including mitotic proliferation of the somatic cells [12]. As a result, there is the formation of the ovarian cavity and spermatic ducts and lobules that will give origin to the ovaries and testes, respectively [9, 13].

In males, it is known that primordial germ cells establish specific positions, depending on the pattern of testicular organization [14]. This pattern, found in adult males, differs between basal (Ostariophysi) and derived taxa (Neoteleostei) [15]. However, the same does not happen to adult females. In this aspect, this chapter will describe the gonadal morphogenesis, with special attention to the formation of the ovarian cavity and establishment of the germinal epithelium, in basal taxa (*Tanichthys albonubes* and *Corydoras schwartzi*) and derived taxa (*Amatitlania nigrofasciata*), verifying possible distinctions or existing patterns along gonadal differentiation and considering the position of the species on the phylogenetic scale. The different methods used for these analyses are described in "complementary material," at the end of the chapter.

These three representatives were chosen because they are small ornamental species, quite resistant and known in ornamental aquarium. In addition, they can be reproduced in aquarium, presenting a fast period of differentiation. Although gonadal differentiation is quick in these representatives, the data showed here can be extrapolated to the species of their groups, since there is no difference in the events along the differentiation. Thus, despite the time of differentiation being species specific, the events and morphological changes are the same [16].

T. albonubes is from China, and it prefers low temperatures. It is one of the smallest known Cypriniformes (3–4 cm) [17]. Among the Ostariophysi, the Cypriniformes were chosen because they are the most basal order, that is, they represent the most basal taxa. *C. schwartzi* is a tropical fish, from South America [17], very important in the aquarium hobby. It is a small catfish (7 cm), and for this reason, it was chosen to represent the other catfish. Catfishes present considerable commercial importance, and many of the largest species are farmed or fished for food. *A. nigrofasciata* is popularly known as acara cichlid. It attains the maximum length of 10 cm. Like other cichlids, it is aggressive and territorialist. Originated from Central America, they prefer alkaline and hot water [17]. Here, this species represents all other cichlids, that is, the most derived taxa.

2. The ovary differentiation in Teleostei

2.1. Gonadal primordium

In Teleostei, as in other vertebrates, the primordial germ cells (PGCs) differentiate from yolk sac cells, originating from extragonadal regions, and migrate to the genital ridge during embryonic development [18, 19]. The genital ridge is formed by a thickening of the intermediate mesoderm, which protrudes ventrally into the coelomic cavity of the embryo being delimited by a mesothelium [6, 18, 19].

The primordial germ cells (PGCs) migrate to the genital ridge and are disposed between the somatic cells. Both cell populations proliferate by mitosis constituting the gonadal primordium [14, 16, 19, 20], as observed in *T. albonubes* (**Figure 1**). Therefore, during the morphogenesis period, the gonadal primordium is formed; it increases in length by mitotic proliferation of its cells, and it gives rise to an undifferentiated gonad [9, 10, 12, 14, 16, 21]. Now, the undifferentiated gonad will undergo a series of structural modifications determining the formation of a female or male gonad.

The gonadal primordia of the species here taken as representatives of the basal (*T. albonubes* and *C. schwartzi*) and derived taxa (*A. nigrofasciata*) present patterns of organization, which are very similar to each other and to the other Teleostei [22]. They are presented in pairs on the peritoneum along the coelomatic cavity, connected by a thin layer of gonadal mesentery. Each gonadal primordium is located ventrally to the kidney and dorsally to the swim bladder. The gonadal primordium extends throughout the entire coelomatic cavity, from the posterior to the anterior region (**Figure 1A** and **B**).

These characteristics of the gonadal primordium are also found in the adult form of the species that present an odd gonad, such as Poeciliids, a viviparous species, considered derived taxa [14, 23, 24]. In these, the formation of bilateral gonadal primordia is common. However, both gonadal primordia merge during the development of the gonadal tissue, forming a single organ in the adult individual [3, 14, 23].

Histologically, the gonadal primordia are formed by primordial germ cells (PGCs) and somatic cells. The somatic cells show varied forms, being predominantly squamous, with basophilic nucleus and scarce cytoplasm. The PGCs are large oval cells with voluminous nucleus and show quite evident nucleolus. Their cytoplasm is scarce and rich in "nüage," presenting positive response to metanil yellow, indicating the presence of proteins in its constitution (**Figure 1C**).

The primordial germ cells (PGCs) are distributed along the gonadal primordium, which is filiform, long, and thin, composed by only one or two layers of PGCs. Mitotic activity of PGCs may be occasionally visualized.

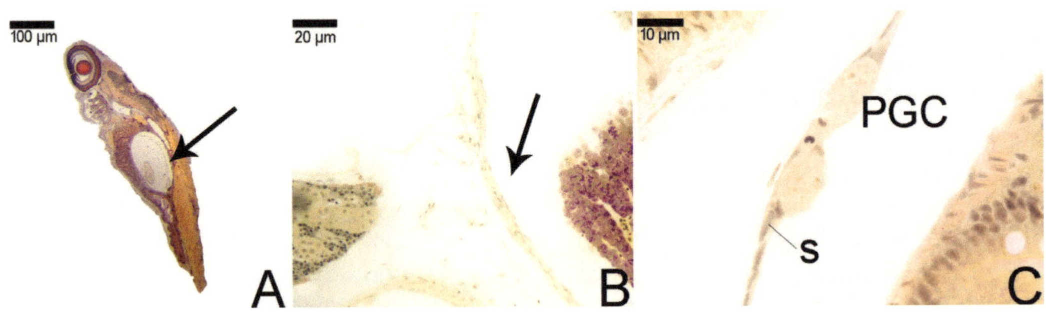

Figure 1. The gonadal primordium in *T. albonubes*. Light microscopy. Parasagittal sections. (A, B) The gonadal primordium (arrow) is located ventral to the kidney and dorsal to the gut. (C) The gonadal primordium is formed by primordial germ cells (PGCs) and somatic cell(s). Staining: periodic acid Schiff + hematoxylin + metanil yellow.

At this stage, in any of the species, there are no morphological differences which suggest the evolution toward a male or female gonad. The number of germ and somatic cells gradually increases throughout the gonadal development. As a result, there is an increase in the size of the gonadal tissue, which becomes an undifferentiated gonad.

2.2. Undifferentiated gonad

The undifferentiated gonads of *T. albonubes* and *A. nigrofasciata* (**Figure 2A–D**) were observed in animals up to 30 days postfertilization (dpf) with 0.5 and 0.7 cm in length, respectively. In *C. schwartzi* the gonads remain undifferentiated (**Figure 2E** and **F**) for a longer period, up to 120 dpf, when the animals measure 2.5 cm.

In these species, as in most Teleostei, the undifferentiated gonads are pairs, long, and thin, occupying two-thirds of the coelomatic cavity from the urogenital papillae. They are formed by primordial germ cells (PGCs) dispersed among somatic cells.

In parasagittal sections, the undifferentiated gonads are thicker in comparison with the gonadal primordium, mainly due to the greater amount of somatic cells, which present irregular and squamous forms. The primordial germ cells (PGCs) remain in small numbers and are initially isolated between somatic cells, scattered throughout the gonad (**Figure 2**).

Since the undifferentiated gonads are formed only by primordial germ cells and somatic cells, they are very similar in any group of fishes, from the basal to the most derived taxa, including primitive fish such as sturgeon [25] or species with indirect gonochoristic development as Cypriniformes *Danio rerio* [26] and Characiformes *Gymnocorymbus ternetzi* [21], both Ostariophysians.

2.3. Gonadal differentiation

Morphological changes in the gonadal tissue, such as the formation of the ovarian cavity and the entrance into meiosis of the germ cells in females or the formation of the testicular ducts and lobules in males, are the main parameters used for the sexual distinction of gonochoristic gonads. Although these characteristics gather the consensus among different authors [6, 13], who use them as parameters for gonadal differentiation, the distinction between the female and male gonads may be detected prior to the entrance of the primordial germ cells into meiosis or before the formation of gonadal structures by the somatic cells. This detection of presumed female or male gonads is possible when considering the organization of germ and somatic cells in the gonadal tissue [14]. In other words, the gonadal differentiation in many species of Teleostei is closely related to the organization of the cellular types, which constitute the early gonadal tissue [14, 16].

A peculiarity observed here in *A. nigrofasciata* is the fact that the pattern of cellular organization in the undifferentiated gonads is different between female and male gonads [14], i.e., early gonads that will supposedly give rise to the ovaries and testes already present certain morphological differentiation. The same was observed in other derived taxa, such as *Poecilia reticulata* [14], being a common feature among the derived groups, that is, Neoteleostei.

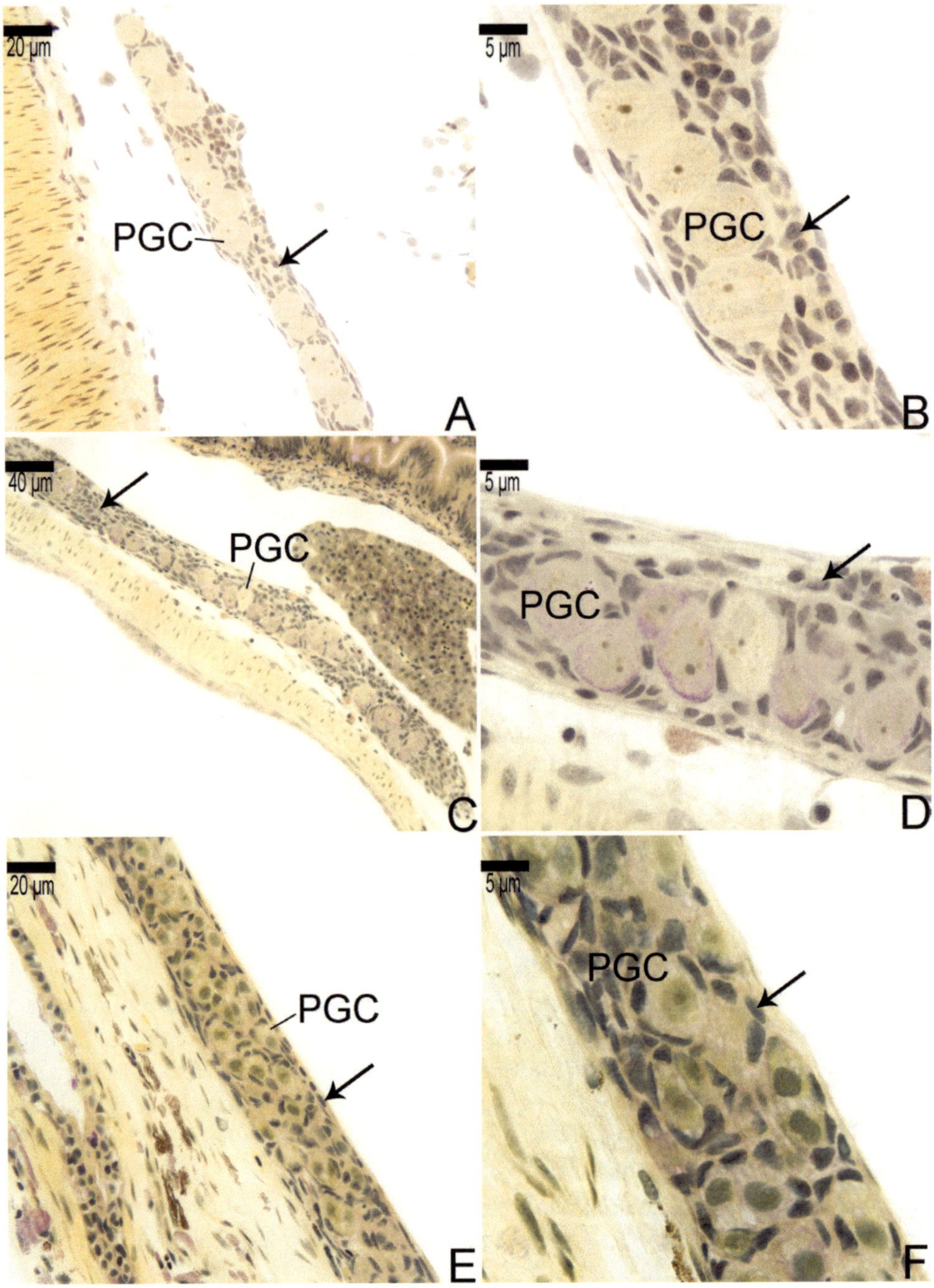

Figure 2. The undifferentiated gonads in *T. albonubes* (A, B), *A. nigrofasciata* (C, D), and *C. schwartzi* (E, F). Light microscopy. Parasagittal sections. The undifferentiated gonads are very elongated, are thin, and show a major number of somatic cells (arrow). The primordial germ cells (PGCs) are surrounded by somatic cells. Staining: periodic acid Schiff + hematoxylin + metanil yellow.

http://dx.doi.org/10.5772/intechopen.69022

However, this pattern of organization of the Neoteleostei differs from the one found in the representatives of the Ostariophysi here utilized (*T. albonubes* and *C. schwartzi*), which present patterns similar to most of the existing descriptions for Teleostei [6, 12, 16, 18, 19, 22, 27].

In these, the supposedly female animals present primordial germ cells distributed in the central region of the early gonadal tissue, which has a smaller number of somatic cells concentrated mainly in the peripheral region of the gonad. At this stage, among most basal fish, it is possible to differentiate female from male gonads. In female gonads, the oogonia proliferate, form continuous cords of cells, and enter into meiosis, originating the first oocytes [16], while in male gonads, spermatogonia are organized in acinar structure or cell clusters, after forming continuous cords [14].

Thus, before the appearance of structures such as the ovarian cavity formation, the female gonadal differentiation in both Ostariophysi and Neoteleostei is initially marked by the appearance of meiotic figures in gonadal tissue [12, 13, 16].

The gonads of *T. albonubes*, *C. schwartzi*, and *A. nigrofasciata* differentiate directly into the ovary or testis, presenting direct gonochoristic development. In these three species, gradually and close to the period preceding gonadal differentiation, there is a small difference in the distribution of primordial germ cells (PGCs) along the gonadal tissue, between the supposedly female and male gonads.

In *T. albonubes* and *A.* nigrofasciata, the ovarian differentiation precedes the testicular differentiation and occurs around 37 and 120 dpf, respectively (in animals measure 1 and 3 cm). In contrast, in *C. schwartzi*, the ovarian and testicular differentiation occurs simultaneously around 130–150 dpf (3–4 cm).

In *T. albonubes* and *A. nigrofasciata*, the supposedly female gonad is smaller in size than the supposedly male one. The ratio of primordial germ cells (PGCs) to somatic cells is more balanced in females, whereas in supposedly male gonads, PGCs are scarce and are scattered among countless somatic cells. As a consequence, the male gonad becomes thicker than the female gonad [14]. Furthermore, in the supposedly female gonads, there is usually only a single line of PGCs delimited by somatic cells due to the gonad lower thickness.

In *C. schwartzi*, the first indication of gonadal differentiation refers to the organization of germ cells in supposedly male and female gonads. In female gonads, the oogonia form small germline cysts, separated by a highly developed interstitial tissue.

As it can be observed in these species, as well as in most Teleostei, the events involved in ovarian differentiation are quite similar, distinguishing between the species only in the chronology and the way in which the processes concurs to achieve the same final result—the formation of a cavity organ delimited by a germinal epithelium. Thus, the first stages of ovarian differentiation, characterized by the entrance of the germ cells into meiosis and the beginning of the folliculogenesis process, did not present significant differences between the species.

2.4. First folliculogenesis

The gonadal tissue of the analyzed species is thin, elongated, and formed by primordial germ cells (PGCs), now differentiated into oogonia, and somatic cells. The oogonia, immersed within the gonadal tissue, may be associated with somatic cells or remain isolated (**Figure 3A**). Isolated oogonia proliferate by mitosis giving rise to new oogonia (**Figure 3B**). When associated with somatic cells, they form a cyst of oogonium (**Figure 3C** and **D**), which originates the initial prophase oocytes, upon entering into meiosis, analogous to what occurs in the germinal epithelium of the ovigerous lamellae in sexually adult females [28–30]. The development of germ cells within each cyst is synchronous, due to the presence of cytoplasmic bridges between oogonia (**Figure 3E** and **F**) and prophase oocytes [16, 22, 31]. Thus, the cytokinesis is incomplete.

Since each oogonium gives rise to a cyst and the cellular divisions begin, different cysts are formed next to each other, giving rise to cell clusters, delimited gradually by a sole basement membrane in formation (**Figure 3C** and **D**). Thus, throughout the gonad, it is possible to observe individual isolated oogonia between somatic cells and cysts delimited by somatic cells derived from the epithelium, containing oogonia and/or early prophase oocytes (**Figure 3G**).

The oogonia are oval cells that present scarce cytoplasm with granulations corresponding to "nüages." Their nuclei are large and spherical with one or more evident nucleoli. Its cytoplasm presents spherical mitochondria with tubular ridges, often associated with "nüages" (**Figure 3A–D**).

Oocytes present in the cysts are also rounded, with nuclei containing chromatin in different forms of organization according to the stage of the prophase in which they are found (**Figure 3G–M**), but their cytoplasm does not differ them, always remaining slightly acidophilus and scarce. Initially, the prophase oocytes have a more basophilic nucleus than the oogonia, and there is a decrease in the amount of "nüage" in the cytoplasm. The leptotene oocyte shows a strongly basophilic nucleus, with at least one nucleolus quite evident. With the progression of the prophase, the oocyte gradually lost nuclear basophilia. The zygotene oocyte presents greater chromosome condensation, giving the nucleus a granular aspect. Formation of the synaptonemic complexes begins, allowing the pairing of the homologous chromosomes. In pachytene, the synaptonemic complexes are totally formed. In the nucleus of the oocyte, there is a strong basophilia next to the nuclear envelope. These stages are illustrated below.

Now, the germline cysts containing diplotene oocytes are invaded by somatic epithelial cells—the pre-follicle cells (**Figure 3I–K**). Pre-follicle cells strongly united by numerous desmosomes complete and gradually involve each oocyte which separates from the cyst, giving rise to an ovarian follicle (**Figure 3L**). During this process, known as folliculogenesis, pre-follicle cells begin to form the basement membrane, after differentiating into follicle cells (**Figure 3M** and **N**). Gradually, the basement membrane is synthesized, individualizing each ovarian follicle. After the oocyte enter and remain in diplotene stage, the lampbrush chromosomes become visible. The cytoplasm of the oocytes increases, becoming gradually more basophilic and initiating the primary growth while within the germline cysts. Now, the diplotene oocyte isolated in the ovarian follicle, and in

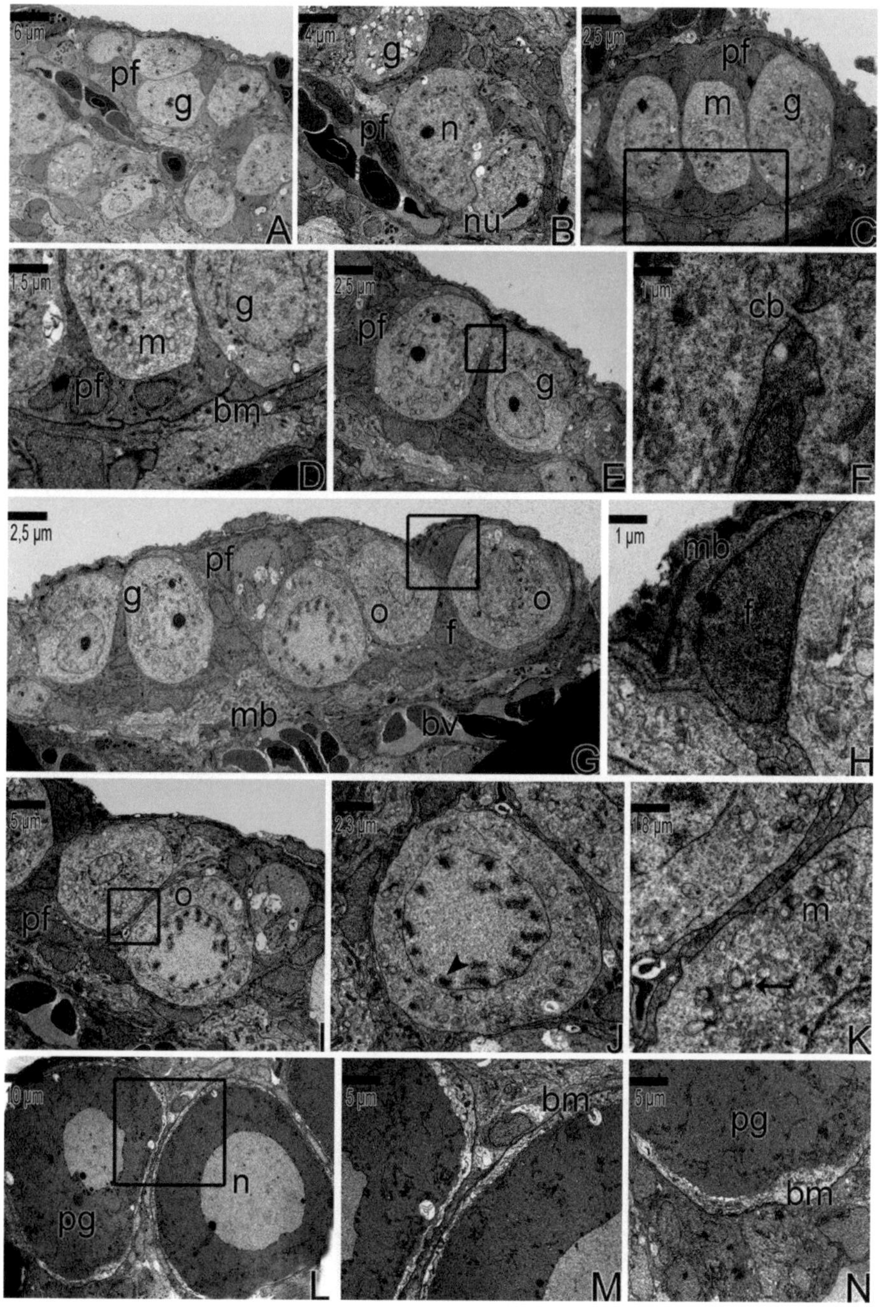

Figure 3. Transmission electron microscopy of *A. nigrofasciata* ovaries, showing details of the process of folliculogenesis. In the gonadal tissue, the oogonia (g) are encompassed by somatic cells, pre-follicle cells (pf), forming germline cysts (A–C), delimited by a basement membrane (bm) (C,D). In the germline cysts, the oogonia are interconnected by cytoplasmic bridges (cb) (E,F). The germline cysts of oogonia, oocytes (o), and isolated oogonia are immersed in the gonadal tissue, separated from the other somatic components by a basement membrane in formation (G–K). After folliculogenesis, the follicle complex is formed around a primary growth oocyte (pg) (L–N). Blood vessel (bv), nucleus (n), nucleolus (nu), mitochondria (m), follicle cell (f), synaptonemic complexes (arrowhead), and nüage (arrow).

primary growth, presents a nucleus with a variable number of nucleoli, which, initially located in the central region of the nucleus (oocytes with multiple nuclei), later become peripheral (perinucleolar oocytes).

In *T. albonubes*, the stage of the first folliculogenesis is quite rapid. Thus, with only 44 dpf and 1.5 cm long, the gonad is still thin, but it already presents diplotene oocytes in primary growth (**Figure 4**).

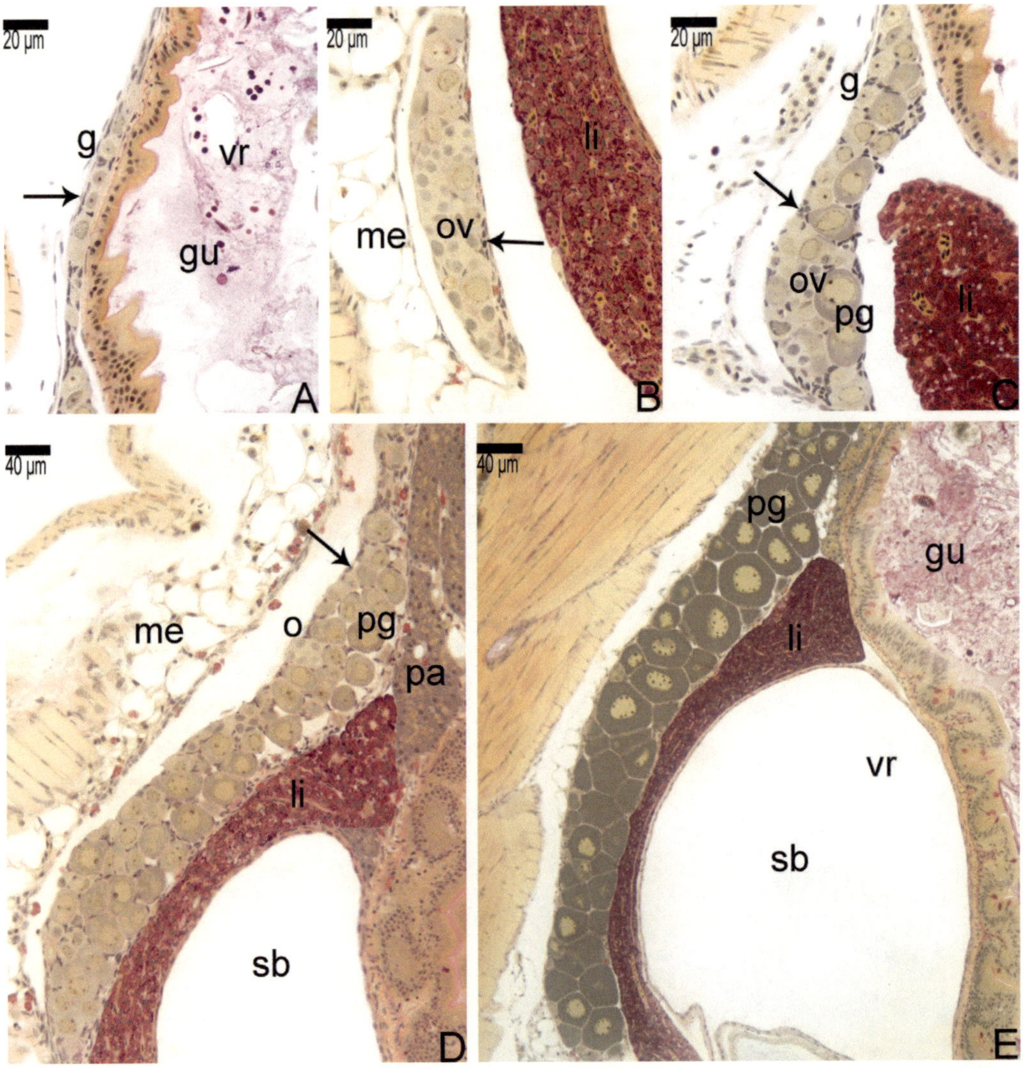

Figure 4. Parasagittal histological section of the female gonads in *T. albonubes* showing the development of the compact gonad, formed by oogonia (g) in A, and prophase oocytes (o) in different stages of the folliculogenesis (B and C). The diplotene oocytes inter into primary growth (D), becoming larger and basophilic (E). Ventral region (vr), pre-follicle cells (arrow), primary growth oocyte (pg), mesentery (me), liver (li), gut (gu), pancreas (pa), and swim bladder (sb). Staining: periodic acid Schiff + hematoxylin + metanil yellow.

In *C. schwartzi*, this process appears to be slower. The gonad remains for a long period, from 130 to 150 dpf, presenting only germline cysts of oogonia and prophase oocytes. These cysts are separated from each other by a developing interstitial tissue, which responds positively to PAS and increases in number, gradually increasing the thickness and volume of the gonad (**Figure 5A–F**). At 160 dpf, in animals with 4 cm, the diplotene oocytes enter into primary growth, but the germline cysts are still predominant, and the gonad is still compact (**Figure 5G** and **H**).

In *A. nigrofasciata*, the folliculogenesis begins after 37 dpf. The gonadal tissue increases in length and thickness (**Figure 6A** and **B**). Oogonia decrease in quantity. Leptotene, zygotene, pachytene, and early diplotene oocytes become numerous and are easily identifiable (**Figures 6C–G** and **7A**). The gonadal tissue presents a large amount of primary growth oocytes and remains with the same histological characteristics until the animal completes 90 dpf (**Figure 7B** and **C**), when presents 2 cm.

At this stage of ovarian differentiation, the gonad is still compact in all the species here analyzed (**Figures 4–7**).

2.5. Formation of the ovarian cavity

In most Teleostei fish, the ovaries are even saculiform organs, presenting a cavity in their interior. This type of ovarian organization is unique among vertebrates and is known as cystovarian ovary [32]. In this type, the ovaries are cavitary organs and present the germinal compartment in the form of lamellae, which protrude from the capsule toward the lumen of the organ. In this case, the ovarian cavity is continuous with the gonoducts [33], which merge caudally and flow into the urogenital papillae [3, 33].

The species utilized herein as representatives of Teleostei have this type of ovarian organization. The constitution of the ovary as a cavitary organ, and therefore the formation of the ovarian lumen, precedes the complete formation of the ovigerous lamellae in all of them, and, depending on the species, it may be concomitant to the constitution of the germinal epithelium. In all cases, the closure of the organ is gradual and can be followed through cross histological sections. Variations of the involved events can occur among the species studied.

In these species, the process of formation of the ovarian cavity follows what has been reported for most of fish [13] and is a result of the proliferation of somatic cells in the periphery of the ovary. This proliferation is responsible for the formation of the laminar tissues, which expand laterally and fuse, enclosing the forming ovary in a cavity—the before-known coelomatic cavity—now, the ovarian lumen.

Despite the similarities found during the cystovarian formation between the groups of fish analyzed, a single divergence could be observed, namely, the location of the somatic cell proliferation regions in the ovary and the direction (ventral or dorsal) of the laminar tissue toward the coelomic cavity.

In the Cypriniformes *T. albonubes*, the laminar tissues grow dorsally to the ovary (**Figure 8**). In contrast, in Perciformes *A. nigrofasciata*, the laminar tissues grow ventrally to the ovary

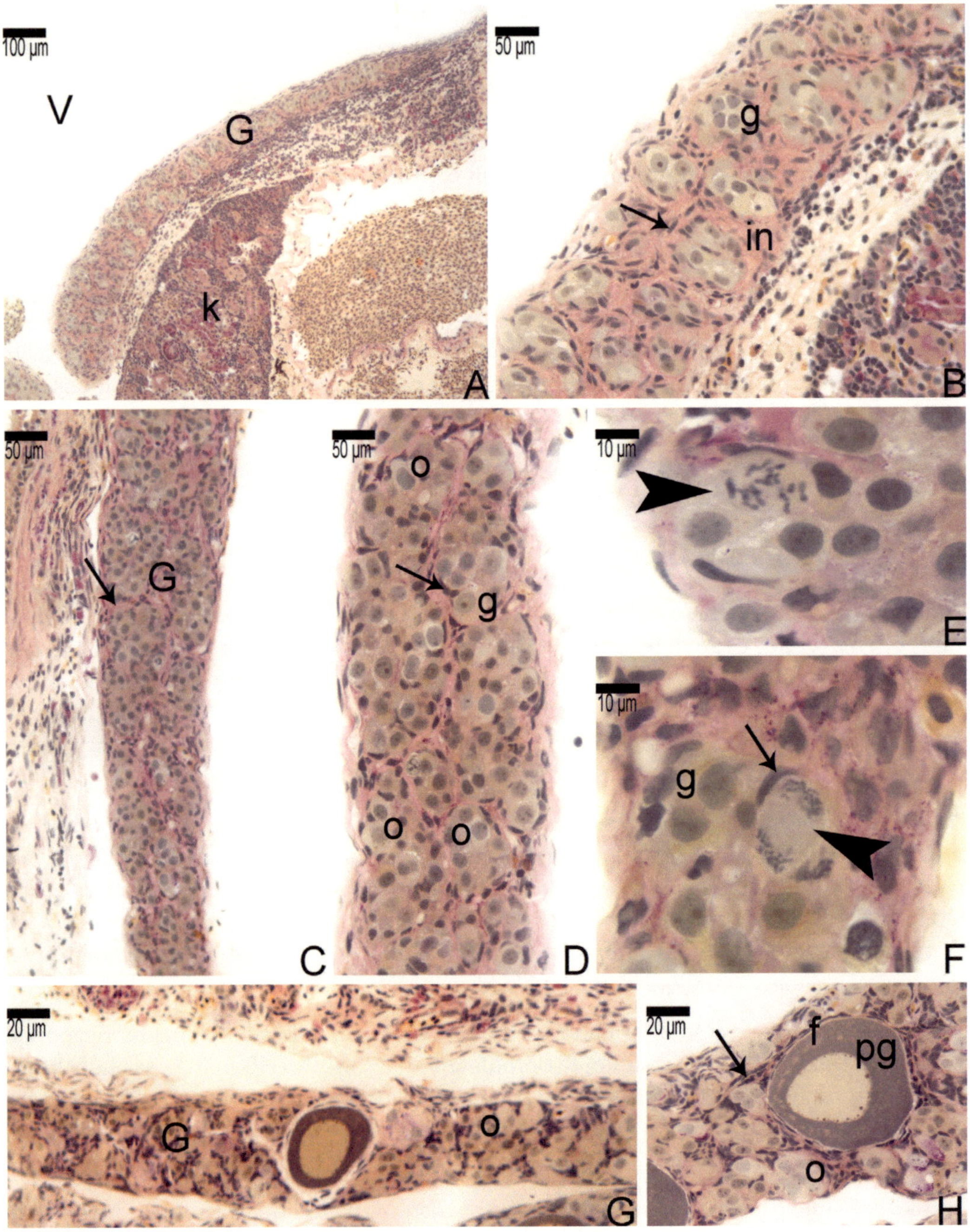

Figure 5. Parasagittal histological section of the female gonads in *C. schwartzi* showing the development of the compact gonad, formed by oogonia (g) and prophase oocytes (o) in different stages of the folliculogenesis. Note the developed interstitial tissue (in) (A–F) and the mitotic activity of oogonia (arrowhead) (E and F). Kidney (k), ventral region (v), pre-follicle cells (arrow), primary growth oocyte (pg), follicle cells (f), and gonad (G). Staining: periodic acid Schiff + hematoxylin + metanil yellow.

http://dx.doi.org/10.5772/intechopen.69022

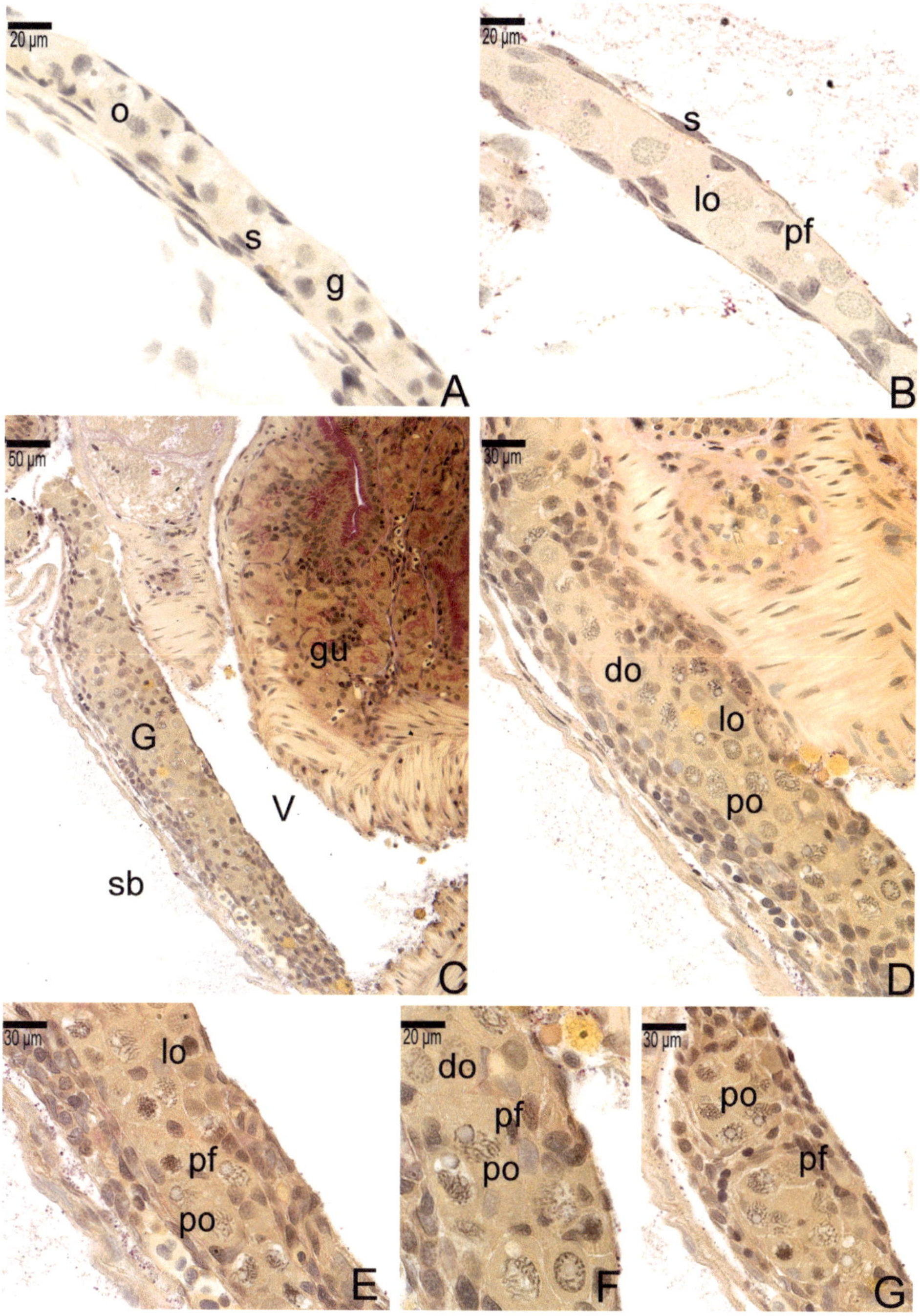

Figure 6. Parasagittal histological section of the female gonads in *A. nigrofasciata* showing the development of the compact gonad, formed by oogonia (g) and prophase oocytes (o) in different stages of the folliculogenesis. Ventral region (V), somatic cells (s), gut (gu), leptotene oocyte (lo), pachytene oocyte (po), diplotene oocyte (do), pre-follicle cells (pf), gonad (G), and swim bladder (sb). Staining: periodic acid Schiff + hematoxylin + metanil yellow.

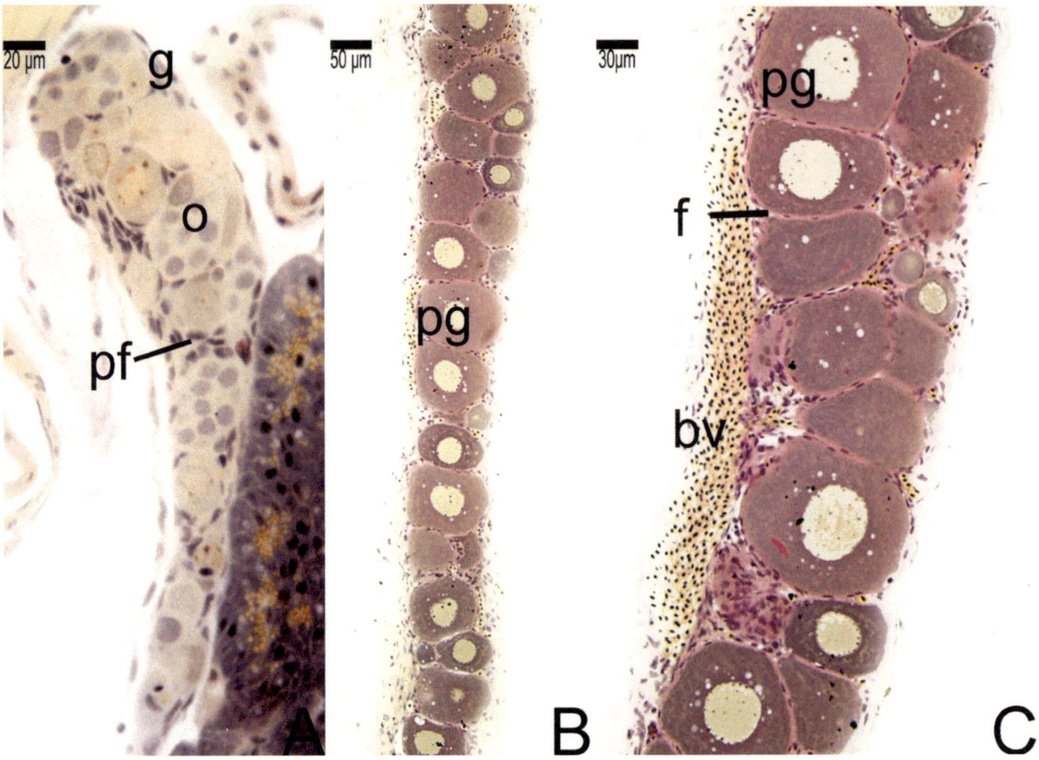

Figure 7. Parasagittal histological section of the female gonads in *A. nigrofasciata* in early development (A), showing prophase oocytes (o) and entrance of the oocyte in primary growth (pg) (B and C). Pre-follicle cells (pf), follicle cells (f), and blood vessel (bv). Staining: periodic acid Schiff + hematoxylin + metanil yellow.

(**Figure 9**), similar to what occurs in *Cyprinus carpio*, another Cypriniformes [16], or in *G. ternetzi*, a Characiformes [21]. Therefore, the direction of the closure of the ovarian cavity seems to vary among species, independent on their phylogenetic position.

In *T. albonubes* and *A. nigrofasciata*, despite pertaining to different orders, being a basal and another derived taxa, respectively, the formation of the ovarian cavity (at 44 and 90 dpf, respectively) is very similar.

In both species, concomitant to the entrance of the oocyte in primary growth, the gonadal tissue, still compact, presents lateral tissue projections from the proliferation of somatic cells in the periphery of the gonadal tissue. Through the cross sections, the growth of the laminar tissue, on both sides of the ovary, can be traced toward the dorsal (*T. albonubes*) and ventral portion (*A. nigrofasciata*) of the gonad (**Figures 8** and **9**). During the growth of the laminar tissues, they eventually find the epithelium of the mesentery in the dorsal or ventral region, in which the gonad is supported. In this way, the laminar tissues fuse to the mesothelium and enclose the ovary in a space—the ovarian cavity. At this stage, oogonia and germline cysts, immersed in the still compact gonadal tissue, are concentrated in the periphery, near the newly formed

http://dx.doi.org/10.5772/intechopen.69022

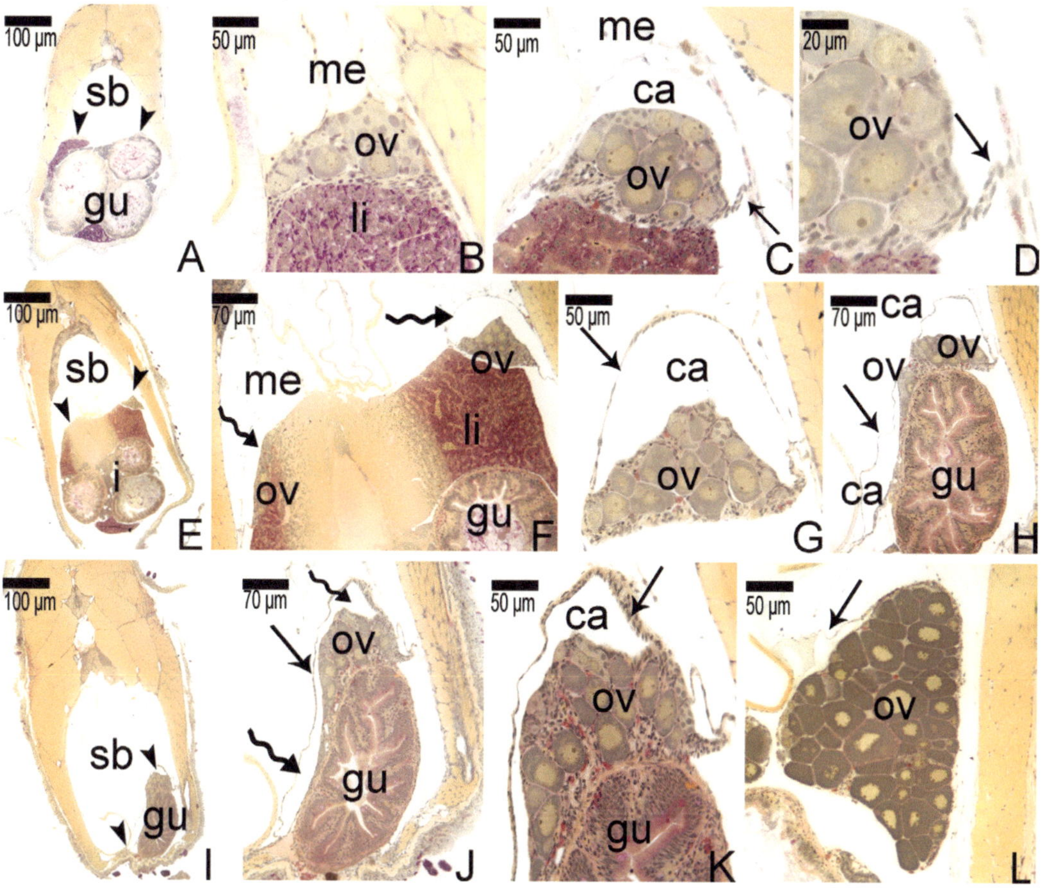

Figure 8. Histological cross sections of the female gonads in *T. albonubes*—formation of the ovarian cavity toward the dorsal region of the gonad. Localization of the ovaries in the coelomic cavity (A). Compact ovary (B) and ovary with lateral projections (C, D). Ovarian cavity (E–G). Note the ovarian cavity separated in each of the ovaries (E, H), forming a single cavity in the caudal region of the animal (I–K). Differentiated gonad with ovarian cavity in the dorsal region (L). Ovaries (arrowheads), mesentery (me), gut (gu), ovary (ov), ovarian cavity (ca), laminar tissue (arrow), swim bladder (sb), and ovarian lumen (sinuous arrow). Staining: periodic acid Schiff + hematoxylin + metanil yellow.

ovarian cavity, whereas the primary growth oocytes occupy the opposite region. This is the first indication of the germinal epithelium formation in *T. albonubes* and *A. nigrofasciata*.

In *C. schwartzi*, another Ostariophysi (i.e., a basal taxa), the ovary is also considered a cystovarian, although the formation of the ovarian cavity occurs by a different mechanism, known as cavitation. In this, the formation of the ovarian cavity is the result of a reorganization of somatic components inside the gonadal tissue, during the formation of the ovigerous lamellae. Thus, in this species, the formation of the ovarian cavity is concomitant to the formation of the ovigerous lamellae and occurs at 180 dpf, in animals with 5 cm. The process will be described below.

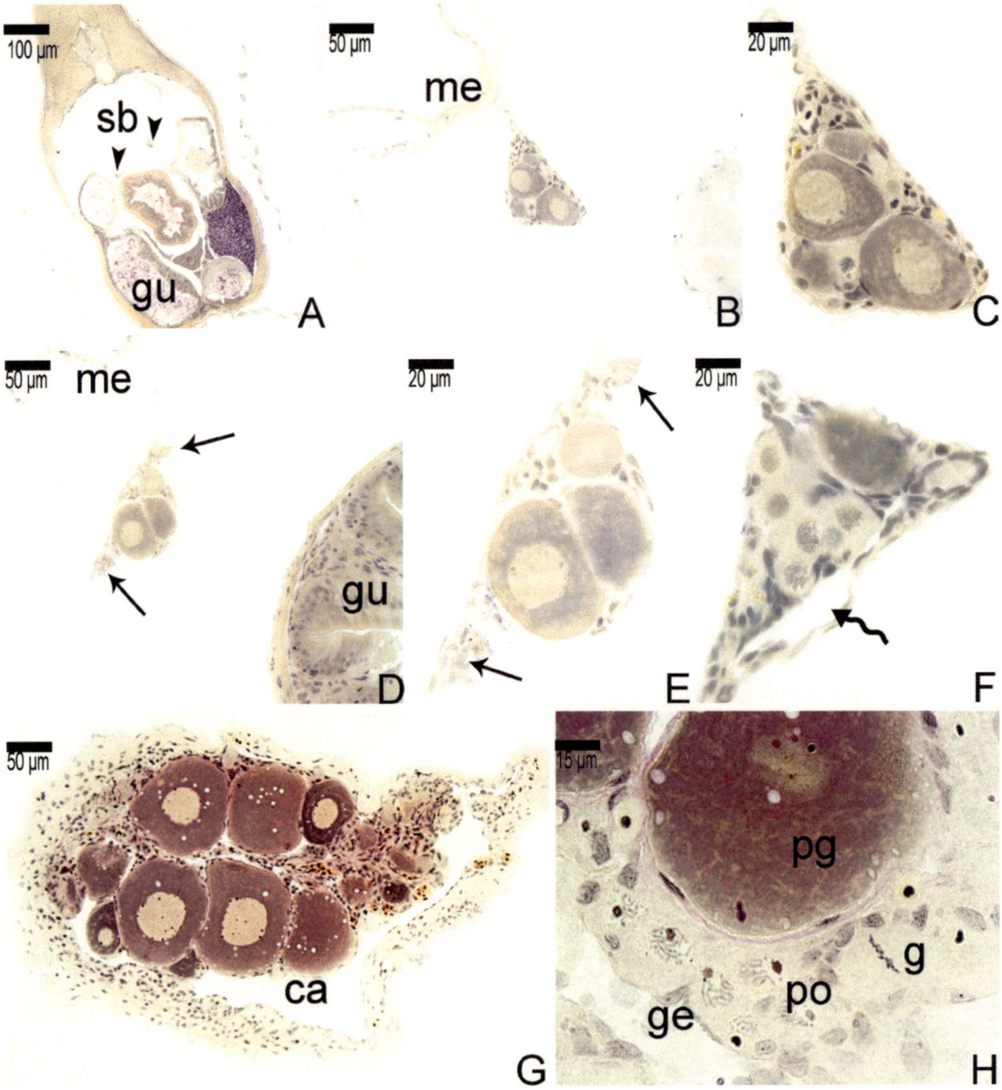

Figure 9. Histological cross section of the female gonads in *A. nigrofasciata*—formation of the ovarian cavity toward the ventral region of the gonad. Localization of the ovaries in the coelomic cavity (A). Ovary compact (B, C) and with lateral projections (D, E). Formation of the ovarian cavity (F) and the differentiated gonad (G), with established germinal epithelium (ge) (H). Ovaries (arrowheads), mesentery (me), gut (gu), ovarian cavity (ca), laminar tissue (arrow), swim bladder (sb), primary growth oocyte (pg), pachytene oocyte (po), and oogonia (g). Staining: periodic acid Schiff + hematoxylin + metanil yellow.

2.6. From the formation of female germinal epithelium to the organization of follicle complexes

In all the species analyzed here, the gonadal tissue is still compact in the stage that precedes the formation of the ovigerous lamellae, even though the ovarian cavity is already formed. In the gonadal tissue, the developing ovarian follicles are gradually surrounded by a basement

http://dx.doi.org/10.5772/intechopen.69022

membrane (**Figure 10**), remaining immersed in the gonadal tissue, along with germline cysts of oogonia, of prophase oocytes and isolated oogonia [16].

In *T. albonubes* with 60 dpf and in *A. nigrofasciata* with 100 dpf, both animals with 2 cm long, from this stage, epithelial cells in movement coming from the gonadal periphery invade the compact tissue forming invaginations that progress into the gonadal tissue, forming interlamellar spaces, which become deeper and deeper (**Figure 11**).

Thus, the lamellae gradually increase in size and project into the ovarian cavity. In the region of projection and formation of the ovigerous lamellae, the somatic cells peripheral to the gonadal tissue reorganize forming an epithelium that borders the newly formed lamellae. This newly formed epithelium isolates the germ cells from the interlamellar lumen. This mechanism, at the same time, forms the ovigerous lamellae and originates the germinal epithelium that borders the lamellae (**Figure 12**) [16].

In *C. schwartzi*, at 180 dpf (5 cm in length), the somatic components within the gonadal tissue undergo some reorganization, resulting in an alignment of the somatic cells throughout the longitudinal extent of the gonad. Thus, in longitudinal sections, there are several double rows parallel to each other and longitudinal to the gonadal tissue, from the cranial toward the caudal region of the gonad. These rows gradually move away from each other, giving rise to a small space that becomes more and more prominent (**Figure 13A–H**).

With the distancing of several longitudinal parallel rows of somatic cells to provide the ovarian lumen formation, the gonadal tissue is separated longitudinally in its central-medial region, becoming pleated. Thus, several parallel longitudinal pleats are formed, each one delimited by the somatic cells that originated them, composing the primordium of the ovigerous lamellae (**Figure 13I** and **J**).

Within each newly formed ovarian lamellae, the oogonia and germline cysts reorganize and migrate to the lamellar periphery, associating with the epithelial somatic cells that compose the border of each ovigerous lamellae, thus constituting the female germinal epithelium in *C. schwartzi*.

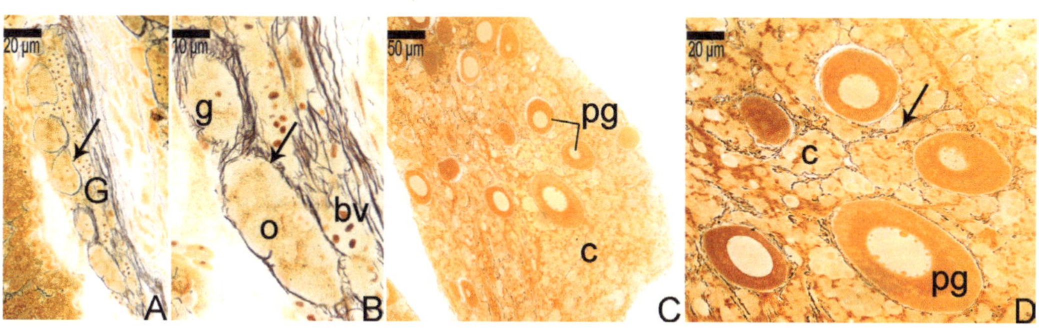

Figure 10. Histological section of the female gonads in *C. schwartzi*—Reticulin method. The germinal components are totally separated from the somatic components in the first stages of gonadal differentiation (A, B). (B) Detail of A. Note the cysts of oogonia (g) and cysts of prophase oocytes (o) surrounded by the basement membrane (arrow). (C and D) After entrance in primary growth (pg), each oocyte is individualized totally by the basement membrane (arrow). (D) Detail of C. Blood vessel (bv), germline cysts (c), and gonad (G).

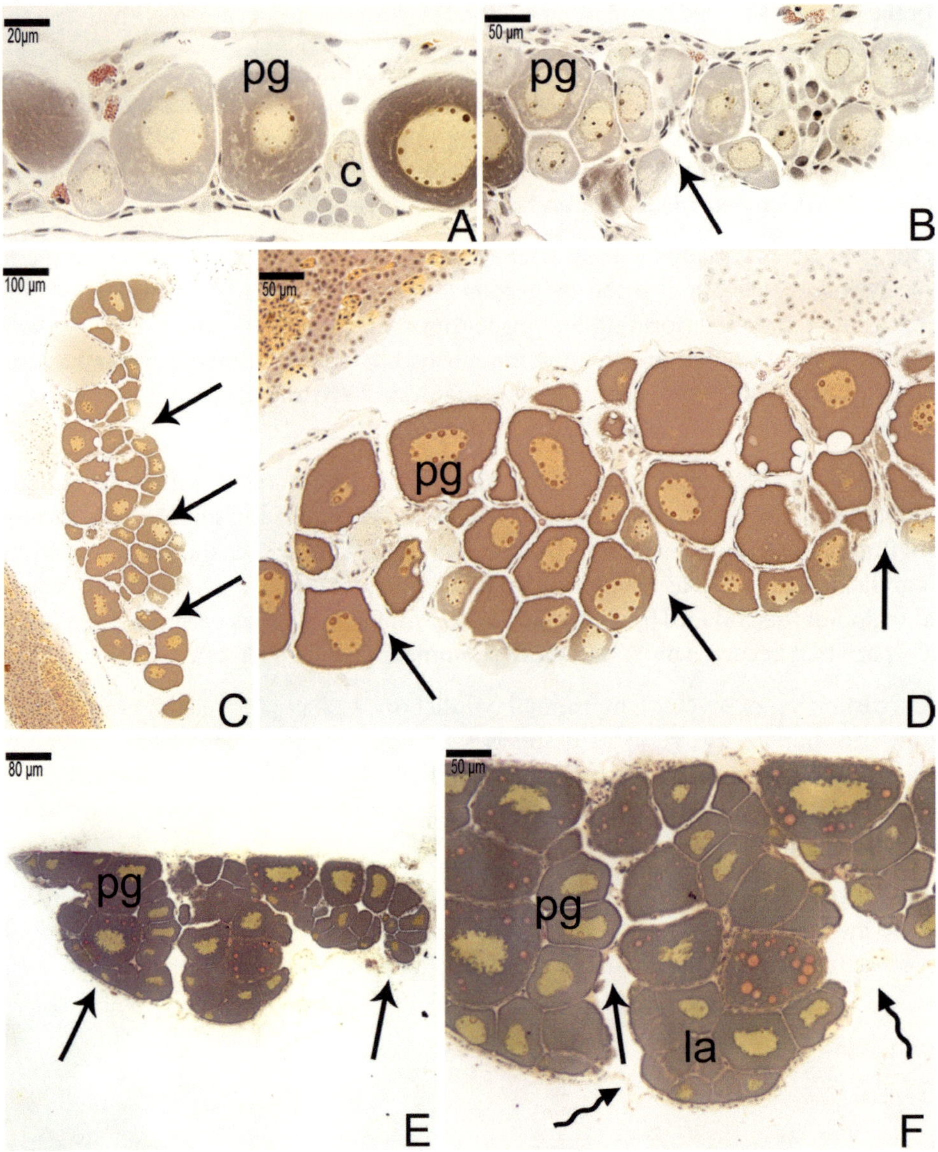

Figure 11. Parasagittal histological section of the female gonads in *T. albonubes*. Formation of the ovigerous lamellae (A–D) and establishment of the germinal epithelium. Ovarian structure already differentiated in cross section, showing ovigerous lamellae in the dorsal region (E and F). Formation of ovigerous lamellae (arrow), germline cysts (c), primary growth oocyte (pg), delimitation of the ovarian cavity (sinuous arrow), and ovigerous lamellae (la). Staining: periodic acid Schiff + hematoxylin + metanil yellow.

By a mechanism opposite to the other Ostariophysi (the Cypriniformes *Cyprinus carpio*), where the ovigerous lamellae arise by the invagination of somatic cells in the gonadal tissue [16], in the Siluriformes *C. schwartzi*, those lamellae are formed by evagination and growth of the gonadal tissue toward the lumen of the ovarian cavity, which is already established. In cross sections, the gonadal tissue presents a little prominent ovigerous lamellae, on both sides

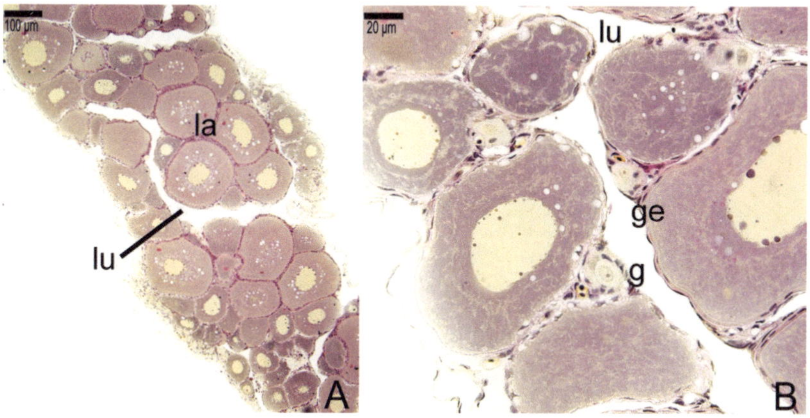

Figure 12. Parasagittal histological section of the female gonads in *A. nigrofasciata*. Ovigerous lamellae already formed (A) and establishment of the germinal epithelium (B). Ovarian lumen (lu), ovigerous lamellae (la), germinal epithelium (ge), and oogonium (g). Staining: periodic acid Schiff + hematoxylin + metanil yellow.

of the ovary. With the advancement of the gonadal development, there is an expansion of the gonadal tissue toward the ovarian lumen, and the ovigerous lamellae become definite.

There are few reports on the different mechanisms that can lead to the formation of the ovigerous lamellae. Therefore, these mechanisms in other Teleostei are still quite unknown, making it impossible for an in-depth comparison along the evolutionary scale.

Thus, even though the formation of ovigerous lamellae is different in *C. schwartzi*, the process that follows for the establishment of the germinal epithelium is the same, even in species which do not present ovigerous lamellae, such as Poeciliids [24].

During the formation of the female germinal epithelium, the somatic epithelial cells, originated from specific regions according to each species, interpose among the germ cells, interconnecting them, after migrating through the compact gonadal tissue. The germ cells, from the beginning of the formation of the gonad, are segregated from other tissue components by the pre-follicle cells. These, in their turn, are supported on a basement membrane. Thus, the germinal epithelium, when formed, will be separated from the ovarian stroma by the basement membrane [16, 21].

In all the species analyzed here, along the female gonadal tissue, there are other cellular components which are interposed to the ovarian follicles already formed and to the cysts of oogonia and/or oocytes. Among these cellular components, small spaces arise and expand gradually giving rise to extravascular spaces. The extravascular spaces are filled by fluids rich in glycoproteins and polysaccharides. In adult animals, they originate from extravasation of blood plasma, which leaves the circulatory system between the endothelial cells and begin to fill regions within the gonadal tissue [15]. It is assumed that the extravascular spaces, in animals with gonadal differentiation, are formed in the same way [16].

Now, this fluid is disposed between the cellular components, moving them apart. Concomitantly, among the cellular components, star-shaped cells with mesenchymal characteristics interconnect progressively, forming a loose network that gives rise to an interstitial compartment [16].

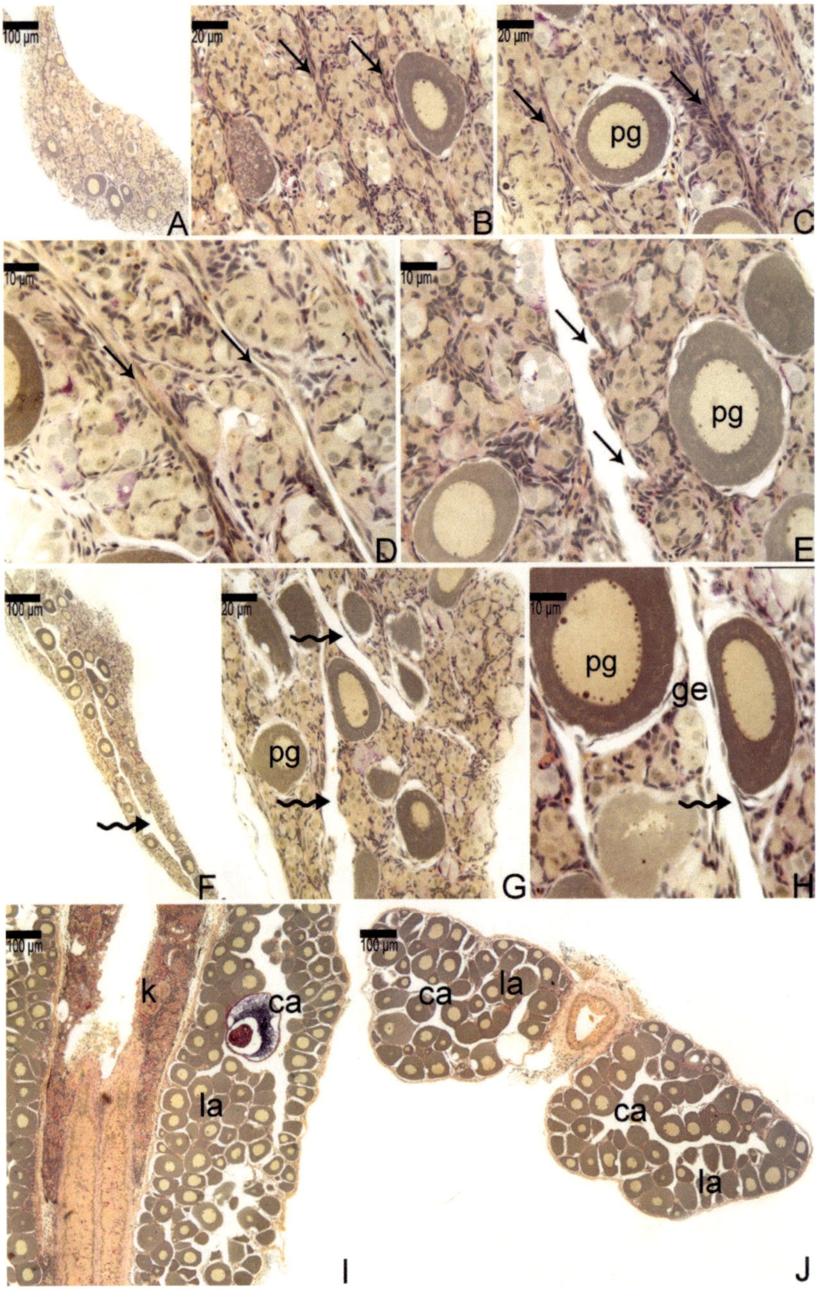

Figure 13. Parasagittal (A–H), longitudinal (I), and cross (J) histological section of female gonads in *C. schwartzi*. (A) Overview of the compact ovary. (B and C) Details of A, showing parallel rows of somatic cells (arrow) among germline cysts. (D and E) The parallel rows of somatic cells move away from each other, giving rise to spaces (arrow). (F) Overview of the ovary, showing spaces within gonadal tissue. (G and H) Note the spaces formed (sinuous arrow) and delimited the germinal epithelium (ge). The ovarian cavity and primordium of ovigerous lamellae are formed. (I and J) Ovary showing ovigerous lamellae (la) with defined ovarian cavity (ca) and established germinal epithelium. Kidney (k) and primary growth oocyte (pg). Staining: periodic acid Schiff + hematoxylin + metanil yellow.

This compartment corresponds to the ovarian stroma, in which new cellular components will differentiate, remaining isolated from the germinal compartment by a basement membrane. The ovarian stroma in the fish is usually formed by a loose connective tissue, in which the extravascular spaces are larger and the amount of collagen fibers is small [16, 28].

From the newly formed stroma, the mesenchymal cells emit cytoplasmic projections which interact with the ovarian follicles and respond from now on by the formation of constituents of the theca. Since the follicles already have a totally formed basement membrane, the mesenchymal cells contacting the follicle, supported by their basement membrane, differentiate into a pre-theca cell and later into theca cells (**Figure 14**) [16].

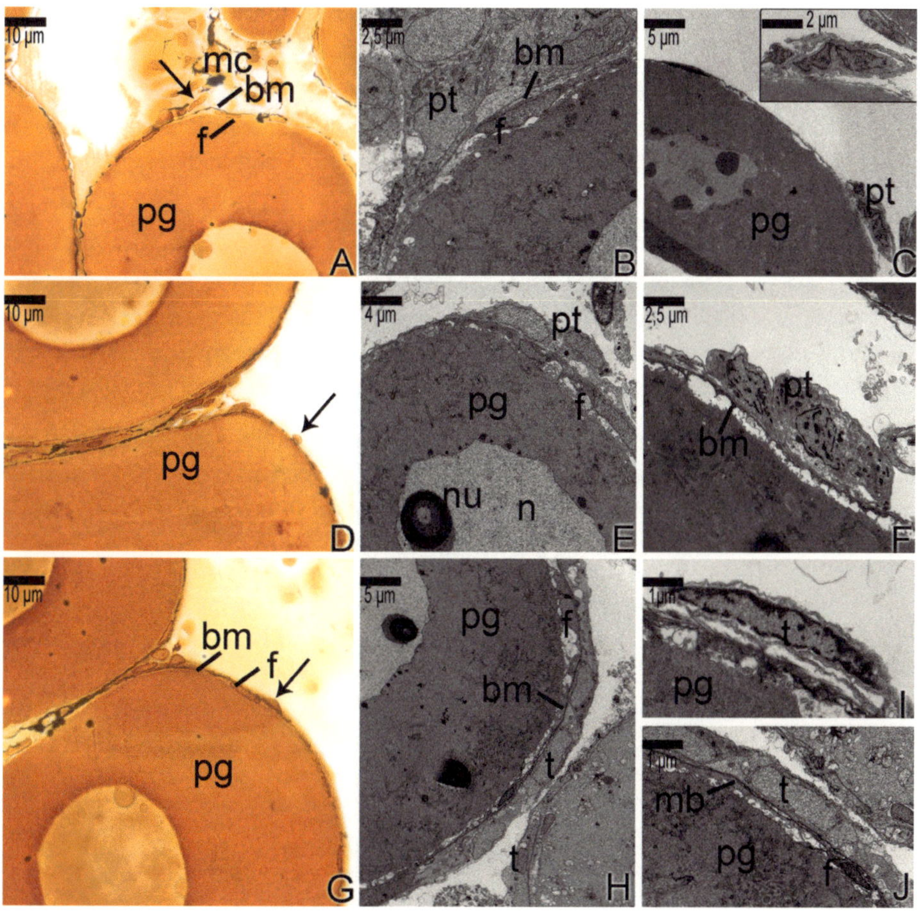

Figure 14. Histological section of the ovary in *C. schwartzi*—Reticulin method (A, D, G) and transmission electron microscopy of *A. nigrofasciata*. Formation of the theca from the mesenchymal cells (mc) of the ovarian stroma. (A) Ovarian stroma constituted by mesenchymal cells (mc), including pre-thecal cell (arrow). (B) Pre-thecal cell (pt) in the ovarian stroma. (C–F) The pre-thecal cell (arrow—pt) approaches the ovarian follicle, and it rests on its basement membrane (bm). (C—inset) Detail of the pre-thecal cell. (G–J) After this process, pre-thecal cell differs in theca (arrow—t) and changes its morphology becoming more fusiform. Primary growth oocyte (pg), follicle cell (f), nucleus (n), nucleolus (nu), and basement membrane (bm).

The ovarian stroma may be more or less developed, depending on the species. In *C. schwartzi*, it presents a developed stroma already in the early stages of gonadal differentiation. In contrast, *T. albonubes* and *A. nigrofasciata* initially exhibit a growth of gonadal tissue, and only in later stages of oocyte development, the gonad will present a developed stroma. Although some species such as *C. schwartzi* present developed interstitial components in the initial stages of the differentiation process, the ovarian stroma is only totally established later.

With the differentiation of the theca cells, the ovarian follicle becomes the follicle complex. The follicle complex is formed by the diplotene oocyte, surrounded by follicle cells, sustained by a basement membrane, and by two layers of theca cells [28, 33–36]. Thus, now the gonad presents two distinct compartments—the germinal epithelium of the ovigerous lamellae and the ovarian stroma [33, 35, 36]—separated by the basement membrane that becomes totally continuous (**Figure 15**).

Within the follicle complexes, the oocyte development proceeds. Microvilli arise in the oocyte plasma membrane and in the membrane of the apical region of the follicle cells. In this region, oocyte and follicle cells contact, and the formation of the zona pellucida begins [16, 29].

Once the germinal epithelium is fully established, it will become permanently active. In the epithelium, the oogonia proliferate forming clusters, denominated nests (**Figure 16A** and **B**). In these, the oogonia associate to the somatic cells of epithelial origin, differentiate, and form a new germline cyst (**Figure 16C–E**) [30]. Within the cyst, oogonia proliferate or enter into meiosis giving rise to germline cysts of prophase oocytes (**Figure 16F–K**). Isolated oogonia, oogonia inside cysts, cysts containing oocytes, and pre-follicle cells start occupying the inside of the same nest [16, 30].

After the formation of the ovarian follicle (**Figure 16L**), the oocyte follows its growth (**Figure 16M**), remaining connected to the germinal epithelium through a certain extension of the basement membrane shared between the follicle cells and the epithelial cells (**Figure 16N**) [16, 30, 33].

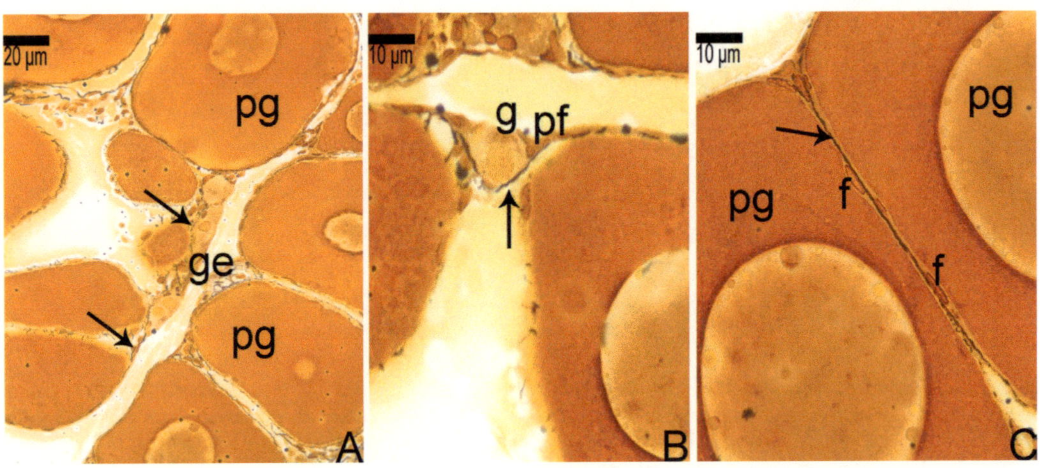

Figure 15. Histological section of the ovary in *C. schwartzi* — Reticulin method. The germinal epithelium is totally separated from the other somatic components (A). Detail of the germinal epithelium on basement membrane (B). Note the sharing of the basement membrane between two oocytes (C). Basement membrane (arrow), primary growth oocyte (pg), oogonia (g), cysts (c), germinal epithelium (ge), pre-follicle cells (pf), and follicle cells (f).

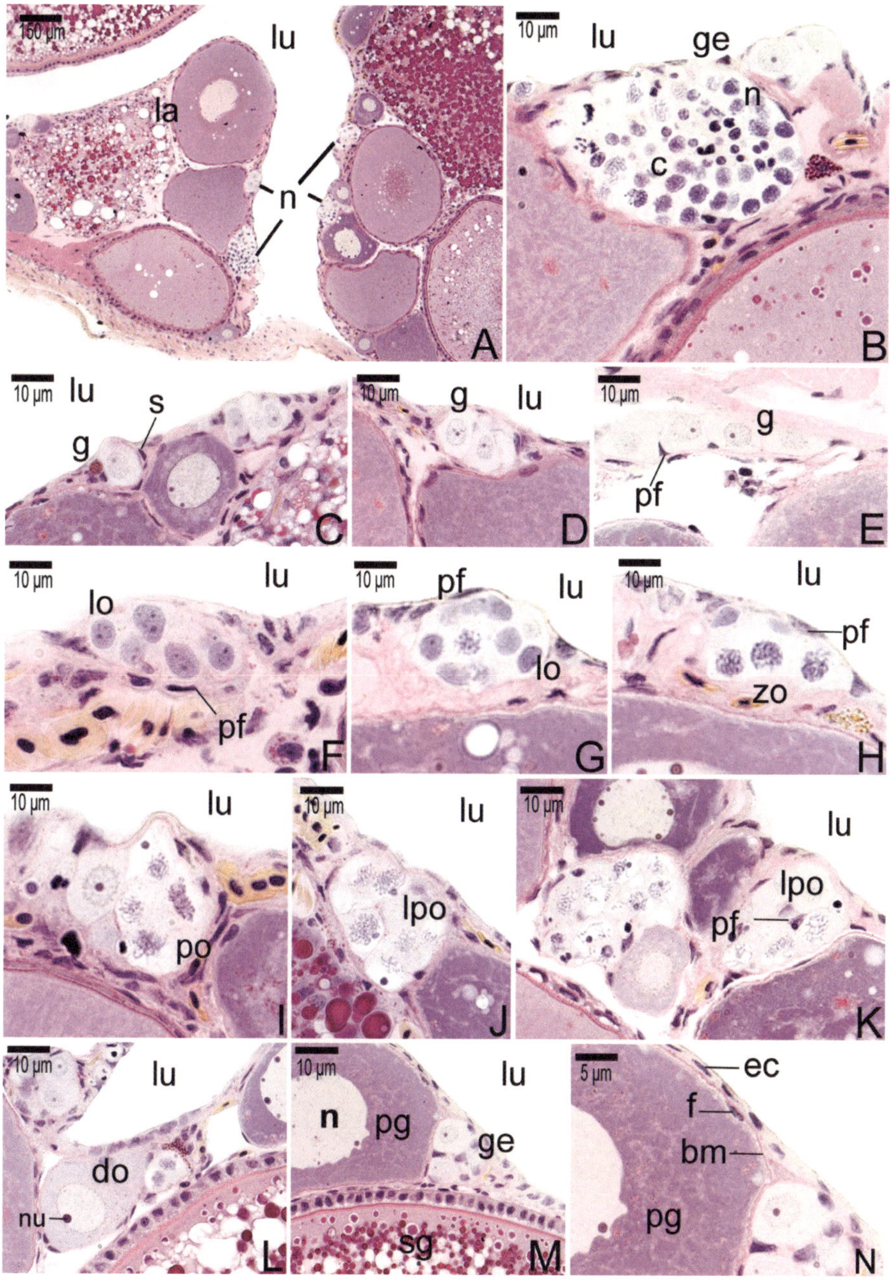

Figure 16. Folliculogenesis in a totally differentiated ovary of *A. nigrofasciata*. (A and B) Cell nests (n) in the germinal epithelium (ge). (C) Differentiated oogonia (g) isolated in the germinal epithelium. (D and E) Germline cysts of oogonia. (F and G) Cysts of leptotene oocytes (lo). (H) Cyst of zygotene oocytes (zo). (I and J) Cysts of pachytene oocytes (po). (K) Cyst of late pachytene oocytes (lpo) with pre-follicle cells (pf) invading the cyst and individualizing the oocytes. (L) Early diplotene oocyte (do) with one nucleolus (nu). (M) Primary growth oocyte (pg) connected to the germinal epithelium (ge). (N) Detail of (M), showing the region of sharing of the basement membrane (bm) between the oocyte and the germinal epithelium. Follicle cells (f), ovigerous lamellae (la), ovarian lumen (lu), germline cysts (c), nucleus (n), somatic cells (s), secondary growth oocyte (sg), and epithelial cell (ec). Staining: periodic acid Schiff + hematoxylin + metanil yellow.

Once the ovarian follicle is formed, i.e., the folliculogenesis process is complete, the oocyte effectively initiates its primary growth [36–38]. From here, the oocytes will be ready to respond to the stimuli that lead to the incorporation of the yolk, and therefore they undergo maturation and subsequent ovulation or spawning [35–38].

The species *T. albonubes*, *A.* nigrofasciata, and *C. schwartzi* analyzed here presented sexual maturity, and they were able to spawn after 180, 150, and 540 days postfertilization.

3. Conclusion

When analyzing different representatives of Teleostei, it can conclude that the processes involved in female gonadal differentiation are quite similar and it is possible to differentiate supposedly female and male gonads, even in the early development stages, independent on being a basal or derived species.

In the three species analyzed here, representatives of basal and derived taxa in Teleostei, the beginning of the female gonadal differentiation is marked by the entrance of the oogonia into meiosis, in early stages of the gonadal development, when the gonad is still a compact tissue. Thus, the formation of the ovarian cavity occurs only after the entrance into meiosis of the oocytes, preceding the formation of ovigerous lamellae in *T. albonubes* and *A. nigrofasciata*. In *C. schwartzi*, the formation of the cystovarian and the establishment of the ovigerous lamellae occur simultaneously. Despite the differences, the folliculogenesis is a very conserved process among basal and derived taxa, with no difference between species.

Thus, although there are differences in the chronology of the differentiation among species of Teleostei, the processes involved are quite similar and culminate in the formation of analogous structures in the different fishes. Therefore, these data showed here can be applied to the most different groups of Teleostei fish.

4. Complementary material

Methodology used: Larvae and juveniles were obtained from spawns of adult of the three species. After hatching, part of the brood was sampled periodically covering the period of histologically discernible sex differentiation. The specimens were anesthetized with 0.1% benzocaine and killed according to the institutional animal care protocols and approval (175/2009-CEEA-IBB/UNESP). The gonadal tissues were fixed by immersion in 2% glutaraldehyde and 4% paraformaldehyde in Sorensen's phosphate buffer (0.1 M, pH 7.2) for at least 24 h.

For light microscopy, the gonadal tissue from larvae and juveniles was embedded in historesin (Leica HistoResin). Serial sections (3μm) were stained with periodic acid Schiff (PAS) + hematoxylin + metanil yellow [39] and with the reticulin method that enhances the basement membranes. Gonadal tissues were evaluated by using a computerized image analyzer (Leica

Qwin 2.5). The reticulin stain [40] uses an oxidizing agent, potassium permanganate, to oxidize aldehyde groups. Subsequently, the oxidized aldehyde groups are detected by the deposition of positive silver ions followed by their reduction using formalin. The result is a black hue of the reticulin fibers. As reticulin fibers are part of basement membranes, the method clearly detects basement membranes.

For electron microscopy, the gonadal tissue from larvae and juveniles was postfixed for 2 h in the dark in 1% osmium tetroxide (in the same buffer). To highlight the cellular structures, block-staining was carried out using an aqueous solution of 5% uranyl acetate for 2 h. Subsequently, the specimens were dehydrated and embedded in Araldite, sectioned, and post-stained with a saturated solution of uranyl acetate in 50% ethanol and 0.2% lead citrate in NaOH (1 N). Electron micrographs were obtained using a Tecnai Spirit Fei Company Transmission Electron Microscope.

Acknowledgements

We would like to thank Brazilian Agencies CNPq (Conselho Nacional de Desenvolvimento Científico e Tecnológico), CAPES/PROAP (Coordenação de Aperfeiçoamento de Pessoal de Nível Superior), and FAPESP (Fundação de Amparo à Pesquisa do Estado de São Paulo).

Author details

Talita Sarah Mazzoni[1,2] and Irani Quagio Grassiotto[3,4]*

*Address all correspondence to: iraniqg@ibb.unesp.br

1 Department of Cell and Development Biology, Institute of Biomedical Sciences, Federal University of Alfenas (UNIFAL), Alfenas, MG, Brazil

2 Institute of Biology, UNICAMP, Campinas, SP, Brazil

3 Morphology Department, Botucatu Biosciences Institute, State University of São Paulo (UNESP), Botucatu, SP, Brazil

4 Aquaculture Center of UNESP (CAUNESP), Jaboticabal, SP, Brazil

References

[1] Nelson JS. Fishes of the World. 4th ed. New York: John Wiley & Sons; 2006. 601p

[2] Nakatani M, Miya M, Mabuchil K, Saitoh K, Nishida M. Evolutionary history of Otophysi (Teleostei), a major clade of the modern freshwater fishes: Pangaean origin and Mesozoic radiation. Evolutionary Biology. 2011;**11**:177. DOI: 10.1186/1471-2148-11-177

[3] Nagahama Y. The functional morphology of teleost gonads. In: Hoar WS, Randall DJ, Donaldson EM, editors. Fish Physiology. New York: Academic Press; 1983. pp. 223-275

[4] Vazzoler AEAM. Biologia da reprodução de peixes Teleósteos. Teoria e Prática. Maringá: EDUEM; 1996. 169p

[5] Le Gac F, Loir M. Male Reproductive System, Fish. In: Knobil E, Neill JD, editors. Encyclopedia of Reproduction. San Diego: Academic Press; 1999. pp. 20-30

[6] Devlin RH, Nagahama Y. Sex determination and sex differentiation in fish: An overview of genetic, physiological, and environmental influences. Aquaculture. 2002;**208**:191-364. DOI: 10.1016/S0044-8486(02)00057-1

[7] Piferrer F. Endocrine sex control strategies for the feminization of teleost fish. Aquaculture. 2001;**197**:229-281. DOI: 10.1016/S0044-8486(01)00589-0

[8] Pandian TJ. Genetic Sex Differentiation in Fish. Boca Raton, FL: CRC Press; 2012. 214 p

[9] Strüssmann CA, Nakamura M. Morphology, endocrinology, and environmental modulation of gonadal sex differentiation in teleost fishes. Fish Physiology and Biochemistry. 2002;**26**:13-29. DOI: 10.1023/A:1023343023556

[10] Yamamoto T. Sex differentiation. In: Hoar WS, Randall DJ, editors. Fish Physiology. New York: Academic Press. 1969. pp. 117-175

[11] Pandian TJ. Endocrine Sex Differentiation in Fish. Boca Raton, FL: CRC Press; 2013. 299 p

[12] Meijide FJ, Lo Nostro F, Guerrero GA. Gonadal development and sex differentiation in the cichlid fish *Cichlasoma dimerus* (Teleostei, Perciformes): A light and electron microscopic study. Journal of Morphology. 2005;**264**:191-210. DOI: 10.1002/jmor.10329

[13] Nakamura M, Kobayashi T, Chang XT, Nagahama Y. Gonadal sex differentiation in teleost fish. Journal of Experimental Zoology. 1998;**281**:362-372. DOI: 10.1002/(SICI)1097-010X(19980801)281:5<362::AID-JEZ3>3.0.CO;2-M

[14] Mazzoni TS, Grier HJ, Quagio-Grassiotto I. Male gonadal differentiation and the paedomorphic evolution of the testis in teleostei. The Anatomical Record. 2014;**297**:1137-1162. DOI: 10.1002/ar.22915

[15] Parenti LR, Grier HJ. Evolution and phylogeny of gonad morphology in bony fishes. Integrative and Comparative Biology. 2004;**44**:333-348. DOI: 10.1093/icb/44.5.333

[16] Mazzoni TS, Grier HJ, Quagio-Grassiotto I. Germline cysts and the formation of the germinal epithelium during the female gonadal morphogenesis in *Cyprinus carpio* (Teleostei: Ostariophysi). The Anatomical Record. 2010;**293**:1581-1606. DOI: 10.1002/ar.21205

[17] FishBase World Wide Web electronic publication. In: Froese R, Pauly D, editors. 2016. Available from: http://www.fishbase.org [Accessed: 22 January 2017]

[18] Otani S, Kitauchi T, Saito T, Sakao S, Maegawa S, Inoue K, Yamaha E. The formation of primordial germ cells from germline cells in spherical embryos derived from the blastodisc of 2-cell embryos in goldfish, *Carassius auratus*. The International Journal of Developmental Biology. 2005;**49**:843-850. DOI: 10.1387/ijdb.052027so

[19] Kunz YW. Developmental Biology of Teleost Fishes. Dordrecht: Springer; 2004. 636p

[20] Kobayashi Y, Nagahama Y, Nakamura M. Diversity and plasticity of sex determination and differentiation in fishes. Sexual Development. 2013;**7**(**1-3**):115-25. DOI: 10.1159/000342009

[21] Mazzoni TS, Grier HJ, Quagio-Grassiotto I. The basement membrane and the sex establishment in the juvenile hermaphroditism during gonadal differentiation of the *Gymnocorymbus ternetzi* (Teleostei: Characiformes: Characidae). The Anatomical Record. 2015;**298**:1984-2010. DOI: 10.1002/ar.23270

[22] Nakamura S, Aoki Y, Saito D, Kuroki Y, Fujiyama A, Naruse K, Tanaka M. Sox9b/sox9a2-EGFP transgenic medaka reveals the morphological reorganization of the gonads and a common precursor of both the female and male supporting cells. Molecular Reproduction and Development, 2008;**75**:472-476. DOI: 10.1002/mrd.20764

[23] Grove BD, Wourms JP. Follicular placenta of the viviparous fish, *Heterandria formosa*. II. Ultrastructure and development of the follicular placenta. Journal of Morphology. 2004;**220**:167-184. DOI: 10.1002/jmor.1052200206

[24] Grier HJ, Uribe MC, Parenti LR, Rosa-Cruz G. Fecundity, the germinal, and folliculogenesis in viviparous fishes. In: Grier HJ, Uribe MC, editors. Viviparous Fishes. Florida: New Life Publication. 2005. pp. 193-217

[25] Vizziano-Cantonnet D, Di Landro S, Lasalle A, Martínez A, Mazzoni TS, Quagio-Grassiotto I. Identification of the molecular sex-differentiation period in the Siberian sturgeon. Molecular Reproduction and Development. 2016;**83**:19-36. DOI: 10.1002/mrd.22589

[26] Uchida D, Yamashita M, Kitano T, Iguchi T. Oocyte apoptosis during the transition from ovary-like tissue to testes during sex differentiation of juvenile zebrafish. The Journal Experimental Biology. 2002;**205**:711-718

[27] Nakamura S, Kobayashi K, Nishimura T, Higashijima S, Tanaka M. Identification of germline stem cells in the ovary of the Teleost medaka. Science. 2010;**328**: 1561-1563. DOI: 10.1126/science.1185473

[28] Grier HJ. Ovarian germinal epithelium and folliculogenesis in the Common Snook, *Centropomus undecimalis* (Teleostei: Centropomidae). Journal of Morphology. 2000;**243**: 265-281. DOI: 10.1002/(SICI)1097-4687(200003)243:3<265::AID-JMOR4>3.0.CO;2-I

[29] França GF, Grier HJ, Quagio-Grassiotto I. A new vision of the origin and the oocyte development in the Ostariophysi applied to *Gymnotus sylvius* (Teleostei: Gymnotiformes). Neotropical Ichthyology. 2010;**8**:787-804. DOI: 10.1590/S1679-62252010000400008

[30] Quagio-Grassiotto I, Grier HJ, Mazzoni TS, Nóbrega RH, Amorim JP. Activity of the ovarian germinal epithelium on the follicle formation and the oocyte development in the freshwater catfish *Pimelodusmaculatus* (Teleostei: Ostariophysi: Siluriformes). Journal of Morphology. 2011;**272**:1290-1306. DOI: 10.1002/jmor.10981

[31] Saito D, Morinaga C, Aoki Y, Nakamura S, Mitani H, Furutani-Seiki M, Kondh H, Tanaka M. Proliferation of germ cells during gonadal sex differentiation in medaka: Insights from germ cell-depleted mutant zenzai. Developmental Biology. 2007;**310**:280-290. DOI: 10.1016/j.ydbio.2007.07.039

[32] Hoar WS. Reproduction. In: Hoar WS, Randall DJ, editors. Fish Physiology. New York: Academic Press. 1969. pp. 1-72

[33] Grier HJ, Uribe MC, Parenti LR. Germinal epithelium, folliculogenesis, and postovulatory follicles in ovaries of rainbow trout, *Oncorhynchus mykiss* (Walbaum,1792) (Teleostei, Protacanthopterygii, Salmoniformes). Journal of Morphology. 2007;**268**:293-310. DOI: 10.1002/jmor.10518

[34] Wallace RA, Selman K. Ultrastructural aspects of oogenesis and oocyte growth in fish and amphibians. Microscopy Research and Technique. 1990;**16**:175-201. DOI: 10.1002/jemt.1060160302

[35] Le Menn F, Cerdà J, Babin PJ. Ultrastructural aspects of the ontogeny and differentiation of ray-finned fish ovarian follicles. In: Babin JP, Cerdà J, Lubzens E, editors. The Fish Oocyte: From Basic Studies to Biotechnological Applications. Dordrecht: Springer; 2007. pp. 1-37

[36] Grier JH, Uribe MC, Patiño R. The ovary, folliculogenesis and oogenesis in teleosts. In: Jamieson BJM, editor. Reproductive Biology and Phylogeny of Fishes (Agnathans and Bony Fishes) Phylogeny Reproductive System Viviparity Spermatozoa. Enfield: Science Publishers; 2009. pp. 25-84

[37] Patiño R, Sullivan CV. Ovarian follicle growth, maturation, and ovulation in teleost fish. Fish Phyosiology and Biochemistry. 2002;**26**:57-70. DOI: 10.1023/A:1023311613987

[38] Lubzens E, Young G, Bobe J, Cerdà J. Oogenesis in teleosts: How fish eggs are formed. General and Comparative Endocrinology. 2010;**165(3)**:367-89. DOI: 10.1016/j.ygcen.2009.05.022

[39] Quintero-Hunter I, Grier H, Muscato M. Enhancement of histological detail using metanil yellow as counterstain in periodic acid/Schiff 's hematoxylin staining of glycol methacrylate tissue sections. Biotechnic & Histochemistry. 1991;**66**:169-172. DOI: 10.3109/10520299109109964

[40] Vidal BC. Histochemical and anisotropical properties characteristics of silver impregnation: The differentiation of reticulin fibers from the other interstitial collagens. Zoologische Jahrbücher. Abteilung für Anatomie und Ontogenie der Tiere Abteilung für Anatomie und Ontogenie der Tiere. 1988;**117**:485-494. ISSN 0044-5177

Chapter 8

The Thalassinidean Mud Shrimp *Upogebia vasquezi*: Life Cycle and Reproductive Traits on the Amazonian Coast, Brazil

Danielly Brito de Oliveira,
Fernando Araújo Abrunhosa and
Jussara Moretto Martinelli-Lemos

Additional information is available at the end of the chapter

http://dx.doi.org/10.5772/intechopen.68934

Abstract

The thalassinideans comprise the infraorders Axiidea and Gebiidea, two distinct groups of decapods that have converged morphologically and ecologically as burrowing forms, commonly known as mud lobsters and mud or ghost shrimps. These groups are an important component of the macroinfauna of intertidal and subtidal environments and are distributed throughout the world, with species diversity increasing from high latitudes toward the equator. These species are burrowing benthic decapods, with more than 95% of species inhabiting shallow waters in marine and estuarine environments, exerting considerable influence over the structure of benthic communities through their ability to bioturbate the sediments, with effects on the infauna and seagrasses in coastal environments. *Upogebia vasquezi* has an ample geographic distribution, it is typically found in rocky outcrops near mangroves. This species reproduces year round, which is subjected to strong seasonal fluctuations in salinity due to the local precipitation regime. The Amazon Macrotidal Mangrove Coast, representing 10% of the Brazilian coastline and encompassing more than 56% of the country's mangrove forests, is a high priority area for conservation. This chapter aims to elucidate the reproductive traits of *U. vasquezi* with a revision about the known ecological information available for thalassinidean species all over the world.

Keywords: Decapoda, Gebiidea, larval biology, reproduction

1. Introduction

The Thalassinidea (infraorders Axiidea de Saint Laurent 1979 and Gebiidea de Saint Laurent, 1979) designates a group of decapods popularly known as "mud shrimps," "mud lobsters," "ghost shrimps," or "corruptos" in Portuguese [1–3]. They are among the most common burrowing shrimps frequently found in high densities in coastal and sublittoral sediments, from brackish to euryhaline environments [4]. Most species are marine or estuarine and use sheltered sites as habitats, preferably estuaries, bays, lagoons, beaches, and seas, both in tropical countries and in temperate regions worldwide, and their distribution ranges from shallow mid- and infralittoral to deeper zones [5–7].

These species are also very sensitive to any type of disturbance in their environments, thus serving as effective bioindicators [1]. The potential to accumulate pollutants in their tissues is higher than that of other crustaceans such as crabs and sand crabs, which is useful in the assessment of coastal environments polluted by domestic sewage and industrial waste [1, 8]. On the Amazon Coast, for instance, thalassinidean species have not been found on coastal sites that directly receive untreated domestic effluents, and have only appeared in less anthropized, more preserved regions [9].

Some species also have indirect economic value, as they are used as bait in artisanal and recreational fishing [6, 10–15]. Its capture is usually performed using "prawn pumps," with consequent trampling and digging in several locations, resulting in relevant impacts to the ecosystems where they dwell [16], as well as on the associated biota [17]. Furthermore, thalassinidean populations might occasionally suffer a sharp decrease themselves or even be at risk of extinction [14]. They have been reportedly used as food in some eastern countries, e.g., *Austinogebia edulis* (Ngoc-Ho and Chan, 1992), which is commercialized in Taiwan [18]. On the other hand, they might also cause harm in oyster farming, provoking sediment instability, that impacts on the growth of cultivated organisms or even cause their mortality [19–21].

Despite the ecological relevance of this species in benthic communities of the mid-littoral, very little is known about its biology, especially regarding reproduction and larval development [10, 22–24], mostly due to its cryptic habit and difficulties in capturing specimens [25].

The aim of this chapter is to provide a brief revision on the biology of Axiidea and Gebiidea crustaceans and characterize the Amazon coastal habitats where these organisms are found, with emphasis on *Upogebia vasquezi* (Ngoc-Ho, 1989), one of the most abundant species of this group in the region.

2. Systematics and morphology

The evolutionary position of thalassinidean shrimps inside decapods is still quite controversial, and this is reflected in frequent systematic revisions. These species have already comprised the Infraorder Anomura MacLeay, 1838, together with hermit crabs, porcellanids, and galatids, among other different representatives of this taxon [26–28]. Although this classification was based on the morphological characteristics of adults, some similarities concerning larval morphology were also observed, e.g., the reduction of a pair of marginal bristles of the telson in the zoeal stage [27], which reinforced indications of a relationship between hermit crab species and this group.

Notwithstanding, important distinctions have also been observed, which indicate a strong association between Callianassidae Dana, 1852 and Axiidae Huxley, 1879 and between Upogebiidae Borradaile, 1903 and Laomediidae Borradaile, 1903 with other Anomurans (**Figure 1**), suggesting a inhomogeneous group [29], which would later be called "nephropoidean" and "anomuran" larvae, respectively [30].

Thalassinideans were later considered a distinct group, at the same hierarchical level as anomurans [31], until they were pointed out as a monophyletic taxon, comprising the infraorder Thalassinidea (Latreille, 1831) [32]. The definition of this infraorder was based on some characteristics shared by the species that comprise it, namely, the complex burrow systems they built and the presence of thick feathery bristles on their second pair of pereiopods [32–34].

However, differences observed between two of the main families that comprise Thalassinidea (Callianassidae and Upogebiidae) suggested that they could have distant phylogenetic origins [35]. Thus, the similar habits between these two taxa (reclusive habits, burrows) would have converged throughout their evolutionary history [35]. This assumption corroborated the indications [28] of the existence of two different groups based on larval morphology. This morphological evidence was supported by molecular phylogeny analyses and resulted in the suggestion of dividing this taxon into two infraorders: Axiidea De Saint Laurent, 1979 and Gebiidea De Saint Laurent, 1979 [36, 37], which has been adopted by several authors [38–42]. Another nomenclature was proposed [43] for these taxa: Callianassidea Dana, 1852 and Thalassinidea Latreille, 1831, respectively. However, the names Axiidea and Gebiidea, which were first proposed by Saint Laurent [44], are the most widely accepted and consistently used to designate the two infraorders, which recognizably comprise thalassinidean decapods [42].

According to the most recent classification [40], the following families are included in the infraorder Axiidea: Axiidae Huxley, 1879; Callianassidae Dana, 1852; Ctenochelidae Manning and Felder, 1991; Micheleidae Sakai, 1992; and Strahlaxiidae Poore, 1994; whereas the infraorder Gebiidea is comprised of: Axianassidae Schmitt, 1924; Laomediidae Borradaile, 1903; Thalassinidae Latreille, 1831; and Upogebiidae Borradaile, 1903 [40]. Since 1792, when the first thalassinidean species were described, currently cataloged as *Upogebia pusilla* (Petagna, 1792),

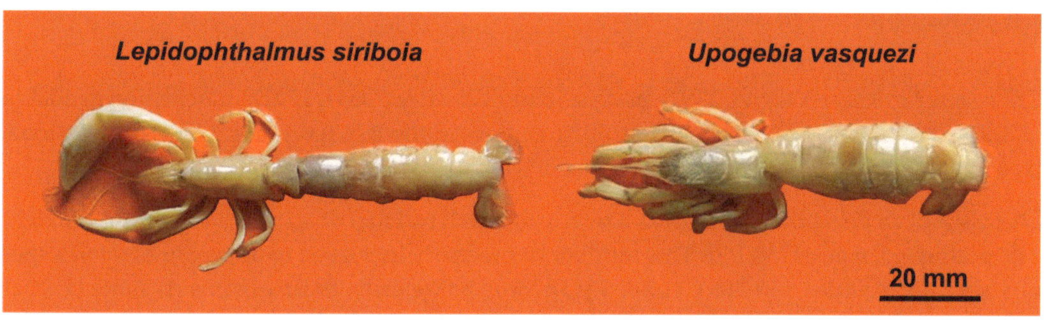

Figure 1. Representative specimens of infraorders Axiidea (*Lepidophthalmus siriboia*) and Gebiidea (*Upogebia vasquezi*) collected in the Amazon coastal region. Scale in millimeters. Photos: Dalila Silva.

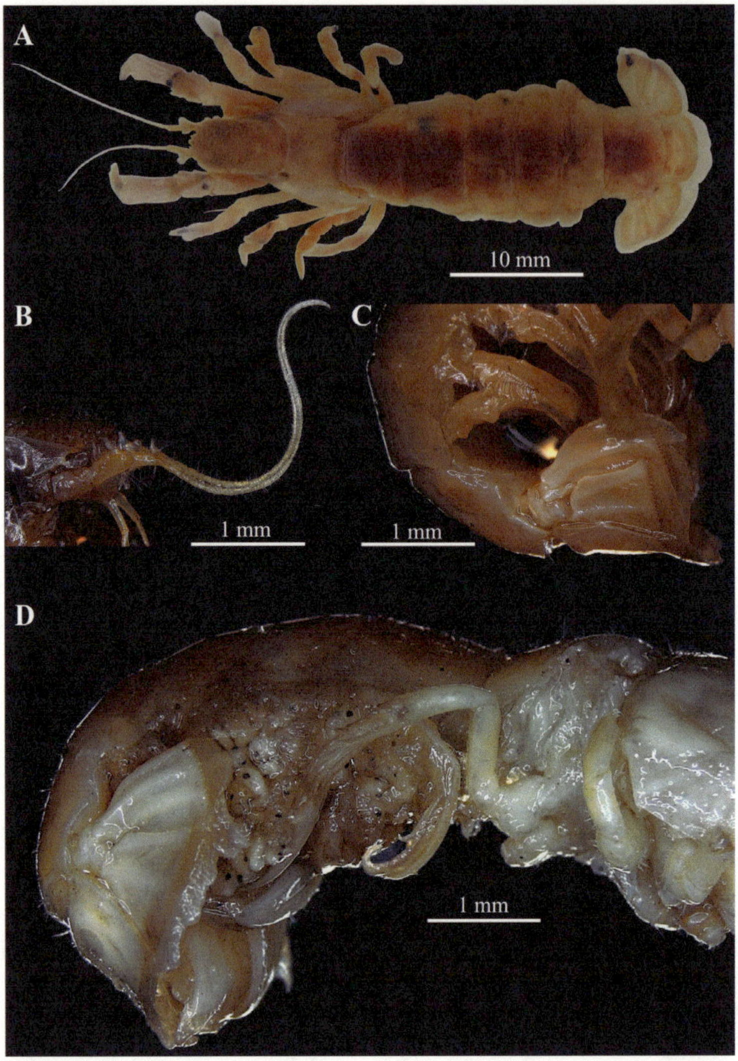

Figure 2. *Upogebia vasquezi*, adult female. (A) Dorsal view; (B) detail of the rostrum; (C) detail of part of the abdomen with pleopods and telson, lateral view; (D) embryos adhered to pleopods in the hatching phase, lateral view. Photos: (A) Rory Oliveira; (B)–(D) Danielly Oliveira.

Callianassa tyrrhena (Petagna, 1792), and *Callianassa candida* (Olivi, 1792), information available on this group has increased considerably, mainly over the last 100 years, and Callianassidae, Upogebiidae, and Axiidae are the most extensively studied ones [7].

Thalassinidean decapods encompass a relatively small number of species, with approximately 646 catalogued species [38, 39]. This number has recently increased to approximately 674 species, with 465 Axiidea and 209 Gebiidea [45]. Morphologically, these organisms share characters such as the presence of a fairly calcified carapace, symmetrical and extended, while the abdomen is feebly calcified, ending on a well-developed tail fan (telson + uropods) [46]. Some species are more similar to lobsters with a highly calcified exoskeleton (e.g., Thalassinidae and Axiidae); while others have a more elongated body and a slightly calcified exoskeleton, better adapted to the "burrowing" life style (e.g., Callianassidae) [45].

Differences between the representatives of the infraorders Axiidea and Gebiidea are mainly the shape of the anterior part of the carapace, the structure of appendages, and larval morphology [30, 47]. Gebiidea have a chelated or subchelated first pair of pereiopods, and the second pair is subchelated or simple (never are both pairs chelated), whereas Infraorder Axiidea has the two first pairs of pereiopods chelated [40]. In addition, Axiidea are frequently heterochelic, as opposed to Gebiidea, whose first pair of pereiopods (chelipods) are of the same size, as can be observed in the two species frequently found on the Amazon coast: *Lepidophthalmus siriboia* (Axiidea) and *U. vasquezi* (Gebiidea) (**Figure 1**).

U. vasquezi has a triangular rostrum, whose lateral edges are nearly straight and longer than the ocular peduncles, with presence of postocular spine [47]. The abdomen is robust, broader than long (**Figure 2A**), and the entire body is adorned with bristles, from the anterior portion, on the cephalic appendages (**Figure 2B**), to the abdominal appendages (pleopods) and telson (**Figure 2C**). Females carry the eggs on the pleopods until hatching, in zoea I stage (**Figure 2D**), with approximately 0.88 mm of carapace length [48].

3. Distribution

Thalassinideans are distributed around the world, with a higher concentration of species in the regions located at low latitudes; e.g., the three major groups Callianassidae, Upogebiidae, and Axiidae occur mainly between latitudes 25°N and 10°N and between 0° and 15°S [7]. The highest percentage of species (36.5%) was recorded in the Western Indian-Pacific, but they are also found in the eastern and western portions of the Atlantic, including the Caribbean Sea and the Gulf of Mexico; as well as in the Mediterranean region [41, 49, 50].

They are mostly marine species, usually found in sheltered habitats, such as estuaries, bays, lagoons, beaches, and seas, both in tropical countries and in temperate regions worldwide, and their distribution ranges from shallow mid- and infralittoral to deeper zones [5–7]. Most species (95%) occur in shallow waters (0–200 m), and few have been found in depths lower than 2000 m [7, 49].

In Brazil, the occurrence of 43 species has been registered [47, 51], and they are popularly known as "corruptos" [1]. Their distribution ranges from Amapá (Northern region) to Rio Grande do Sul (Southern Region) in different habitats, such as bottoms of calcareous waters, coral reefs, rocks, sand, mud, near seaweed meadows, surrounding mangrove vegetation, and in deeper waters on the continental shelf and slope, down to a depth of 820 m [47].

Species of only two families have occurred on the Amazon coast: Callianassidae (Axiidea) and Upogebiidae (Gebiidea) [47], typically found in very shallow waters (down to a depth of 2 m) of estuarine regions with decreased salinity [7, 47]. Only 13 species has been recorded in the State of Pará [47, 52, 53] Brazil (**Table 1**).

Infraorder	Family	Gender	Species	Geographical distribution
Gebiidea (De Saint Laurent, 1979)	Upogebiidae Borradaile, 1903	*Upogebia* (Leach, 1814)	*U. acanthura* (Coelho, 1973)	Western Atlantic: Gulf of Mexico and the Bahamas, Antilles, northern South America and Brazil – from Pará to Pernambuco and along Espírito Santo.
			U. brasiliensis (Holthuis, 1956)	Western Atlantic: Belize, French Guiana, Suriname, and Brazil – from Pará to Santa Catarina.
			U. marina (Coelho, 1973)	Western Atlantic: Venezuela and Brazil – from Pará to São Paulo.
			U. paraffinis (Williams, 1993)	Western Atlantic: Brazil – Pará and from Ceará to Paraná.
			U. vasquezi (Ngoc-Ho, 1989)	Western Atlantic: south of Florida, Bahamas, Central America, Antilles, Venezuela, and Brazil – from Pará and Maranhão to São Paulo.
Axiidea (De Saint Laurent, 1979)	Callianassidae (Dana, 1852)	*Corallianassa* Manning, 1987	*C. longiventris* (A. Milne Edwards, 1870)	Western Atlantic: Florida, Bermuda, Antilles, and Brazil – Rocas, and from Pará to Pernambuco.
		Cheramus Bate, 1888	*C. marginatus* (Rathbun, 1901)	Western Atlantic: Florida, Antilles, and Brazil – from Amapá to Rio de Janeiro.
		Callichirus (Stimpson, 1866)	*C. major* (Say, 1818)	Western Atlantic: North Carolina to Florida, Gulf of Mexico, Venezuela and Brazil – Rio Grande do Norte, Pernambuco, and from Bahia to Santa Catarina.
		Lepidophthalmus (Holmes, 1904)	*L. siriboia* (Felder and Rodrigues, 1993)	Western Atlantic: Florida, Gulf of Mexico, Antilles, and Brazil – from Pará to Bahia.
		Neocallichirus (Sakai, 1988)	*N. grandimana* (Gibbes, 1850)	Western Atlantic: Florida, Gulf of Mexico, Bermuda, Antilles, and South America, and Brazil – from Pará to Bahia.
		Sergio (Manning and Lemaitre, 1994)	*S. guara* (Rodrigues, 1971)	Western Atlantic: Brazil – from Pará to São Paulo.
		Marcusiaxius (Rodrigues and Carvalho, 1972)	*M. lemoscastroi* (Rodrigues and Carvalho, 1972)	Western Atlantic: Central America, Colombia, Venezuela, and Brazil – Amapá, Pará, and Ceará.
		Dawsonius (Manning and Felder, 1991)	*D. latispinus* (Dawson, 1967)	Western Atlantic: Florida and Brazil – from Amapá to Alagoas.

Table 1. Geographical distribution of thalassinidean species (Gebiidea and Axiidea), with occurrence registered on the coast of Pará.

The distribution of *U. vasquezi* encompasses the Western Atlantic, ranging from Florida and several islands in the Caribbean Sea region (such as Aruba and Bonaire), through Central America, Bahamas, Dominican Republic, Barbuda, Antigua, Barbados, Tobago, Mexico, Panama, Venezuela, to Brazil: from Pará to São Paulo [47, 50, 53, 54] (**Figure 3**). It occurs in shallow waters, mostly down to depths of 2 m [7], dwelling in burrows excavated in the sediment of the intertidal zone [47].

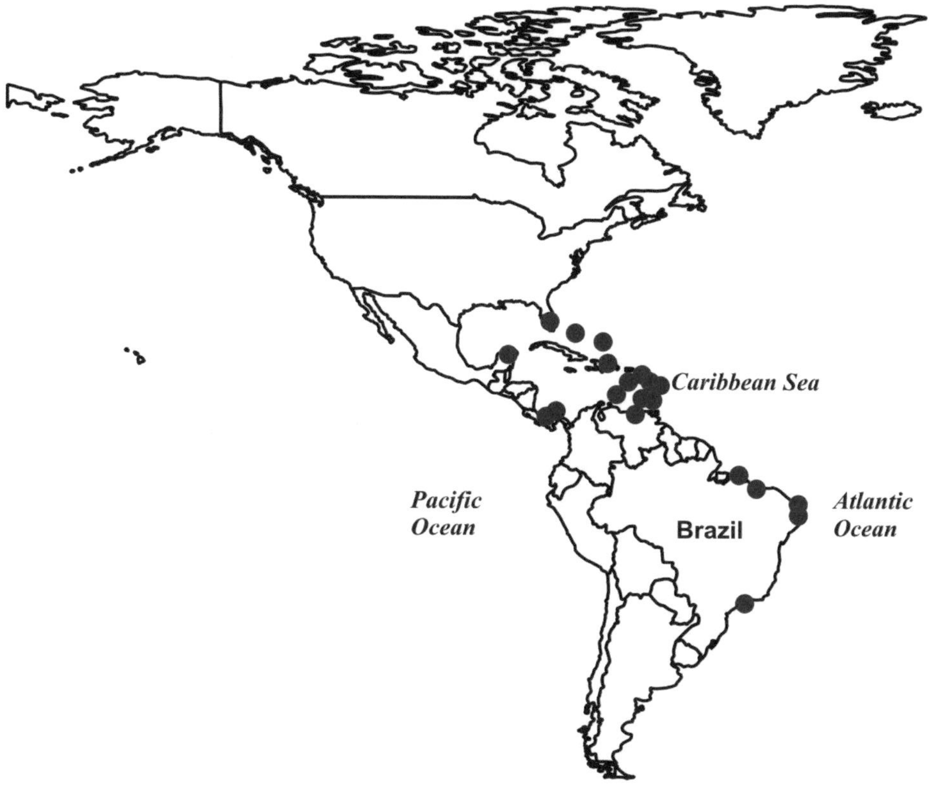

Figure 3. Distribution of *Upogebia vasquezi* in the American continent, according to occurrence records available in references [47, 50, 53, 54].

4. Amazon coastal habitats

The coast of Pará accounts for 6.6% of the Brazilian coast, and the extension of mangrove area covers approximately 2176 km^2 [55] in the northeastern portion of the state alone, corresponding to 1.2% of the global mangrove area (181,000 km^2) [55–57]. The region known as "Amazon Macrotidal Mangrove Coast" extends from Marajó Bay (PA) to São José Bay (MA), totalling 650 km of coast [55]. It is characterized by a wide coastal plain and an extensive adjacent continental shelf (~200 km wide), which is irregular and cut through by several estuaries [55]. This region is subjected to a quite dynamic tidal regime and currents, with semidiurnal macrotides ranging from 4 to 7.5 m of amplitude [48, 55, 58].

Several habitats comprise the Amazon coast, e.g., sandy beaches and estuaries, temporary tide pools, muddy coastal plains, and rocky outcrops, where several decapod species are found, including thalassinideans. For instance, *L. siriboia* occurs mostly on beaches with sandy-muddy sediment [9, 59], *Callichirus major* might be found in habitats similar to *L. siriboia*, on the most exposed portion of the beach (Danielly B. Oliveira, personal observation), whereas *U. vasquezi* inhabits burrows sheltered under rocky outcrops with sandy-muddy sediment [48, 53].

5. Burrows

One of the characteristics shared by thalassinidean shrimps is their reclusive lifestyle, with the construction of burrows, which are among the deepest and most complex systems recorded in transitional marine environments [6]. They are built on sandy and muddy surfaces of the coastal zone, serving as shelter and protection against predators, as well as feeding and reproduction sites [1, 6, 25]. Thanks to the fossilization of burrows on these species, paleontologists gathered important indications about ancient coastlines [6].

Thalassinidean burrows are considered unique environments, whose physical-chemical conditions are strongly influenced by the behavior of these species, mostly due to their bioturbation activities, which have effects on nutrient cycling (for example, see [60–62]) and also ensure high availability of dissolved oxygen, aside from providing protection from the direct action of waves [1]. The process of burrow construction increases the inner surface area of the sediment, in the oxygenated water-sediment interface [33, 63], and causes physicochemical changes, thus increasing the metabolic activity in the sediment [64].

In regions with intense thalassinidean aggregations, there is a change in the sediment structure, which becomes more porous and has increased concentration of smaller particles and organic matter [65]. Such conditions influence the structure of the local benthic community [66], creating, changing, and maintaining a mosaic of habitats for a wide range of organisms [67].

Burrow structure is specific for each species, and it is related to their feeding mode, as well as to environmental conditions and the population density of these crustaceans in their habitats [63]. Externally, they might be divided into two main types: burrows with and without sediment heaps around their openings [63]. Regarding shape, they might be built in a single U- or Y-shaped tunnel, or in several sediment layers or branched, deep tunnels [63], which might be interconnected and might shelter at least one specimen [68].

Most *Upogebia* species, for example, live in relatively shallow, U-shaped burrows, e.g., *U. africana* (Ortmann, 1894) [69], *U. stellata* (Montagu, 1808) and *U. deltaura* (Leach, 1815) [70], *U. tipica* (Nardo, 1869) [71] *U. noronhensis* (Fausto-Filho, 1969) [23] *U. major* (De Haan, 1841) [66] and *U. vasquezi* [72]). Some species of this group build Y-shaped burrows in sandy-muddy habitats, like *U. omissa* (Gomes Corrêa, 1968), *U. yokoyai* (Makarov, 1938), and *U. carinicauda* (Stimpson, 1860) [25, 73, 74].

Burrows of *U. vasquezi* are built in predominantly sandy-muddy sediment, with small and abundant rock fragments, located below extensive outcrops comprised of rocks of several sizes. These outcrops are located near mangroves on some Amazon estuarine beaches, and are submerged during high tide and exposed during low tide (Danielly B. Oliveira, personal observation). Regarding its morphology, the burrows of *U. vasquezi* are relatively shallow and U-shaped [72], and in its natural habitat, it is possible to observe the opening of the burrows excavated in the sediment by just removing some rocks from the outcrop (Danielly B. Oliveira, personal observation).

6. Ecological relationships

Several organisms associated to thalassinideans occur inside their burrows, using them as shelter and also for feeding. Examples are some alpheid shrimp species, as *Leptalpheus axianassae* (Dworschak and Coelho, 1999), the crabs *Pinnixa gracilipes* (Coelho, 1997); *Pinnixa transversalis* (H. MilneEdwards and Lucas, 1842); and *Austinixa aidae* (Righi, 1967), as well as invertebrates phoronids, polychaetes, nemertins, copepods, and gobiidae fish [20, 68, 75–80]. Some species might be parasitic to thalassinideans; e.g., isopods are prevalent ectoparasites of *Upogebia* (Leach, 1814) (for example, see [4, 5, 81–83]). There are also endoparasites of thalassinids, such as trematode cysts, Acanthocephala [4], and copepods infesting gills, pereiopods, and egg masses (e.g., [68]).

In addition to these species, there is a varying fauna that coexists in the sandy and muddy plains inhabited by thalassinideans, not necessarily inside the burrows, which are also influenced by the dynamics of "corruptos" (mud crabs). For example, gastropods, bivalves, echiura, echinodermata, polychaetes, and anemones comprise of an important fraction of the macrozoobenthos biomass in *Upogebia issaeffi* habitats (Balss, 1913) [84]. Stomatopods species, bivalves, and echiura, along with other sympratic thalassinids (e.g., *Upogebia* sp. and *Lepidophthalmus* sp.) [80], are macrofauna also associated to habitats of *Axianassa australis* (Rodrigues and Shimizu, 1992) on the tropical beaches of the Brazilian coast [80].

The invading intertidal fish species *Omobranchus punctatus* (Valenciennes, 1836) (Osteichthyes: Blenniidae) and the shrimp *Alpheus estuariensis* (Christoffersen, 1984) (**Figure 4**) have been

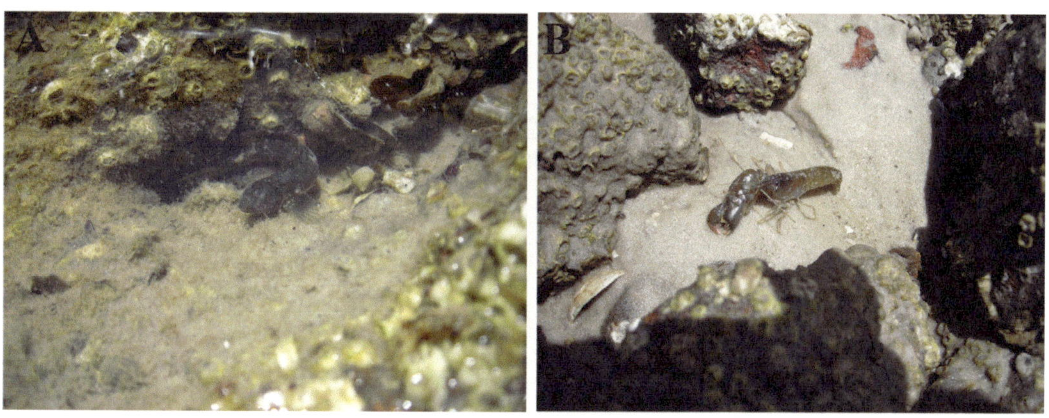

Figure 4. Species inhabiting burrows of *Upogebia vasquezi* in the Amazon estuarine region. (A) *Omobranchus punctatus*; (B) *Alpheus estuariensis*. Photos: Rory Oliveira.

found in burrows of *U. vasquezi* on the Amazon coast (Danielly B. Oliveira, personal observation). Gobbidea fish are common dwellers of burrows of Upogebiidea, feeding mostly on small crustaceans [85].

7. Reproduction and life cycle

7.1. Larval biology

Information available on larval biology of thalassinidean shrimps (infraorders Axiidea and Gebiidea) is relatively scarce, mainly because the development of larval stages of most species have not yet been described, thereby hindering the identification of specimens captured in natural environments. Among the available descriptions, many of them are based on specimens collected in zooplankton samples, which might mislead species identification [86], and in others, the characterization of the different development stages [63] are frequently poorly understood.

Only 12.5% of thalassinidean species and 25% of thalassinidean genera are estimated to have a known larval development, and *Upogebia* is the group with the highest number of species whose larvae have been described [87]. In absolute numbers, approximately 80 species (including unidentified morphotypes of some genera) have had their larval cycle partially or completely described [87]. Some of these species have also had their post-larval stage (or first juvenile stage) morphologically described (e.g., *Upogebia affinis* (Say, 1818): [88]; *U. paraffinis* (Williams, 1993): [89]; *L. siriboia*: [90]).

Regarding the 13 thalassinidean species whose occurrence in the Amazon coastal region has been recorded, only four have already had their larval and/or juvenile development stages partially or completely described: *C. major*, *L. siriboia*, *U. paraffinis*, and *U. vasquezi* (**Table 2**).

The larval phase of thalassinideans is predominantly planktonic, and in most species, it is the only life-cycle stage where they remain outside their burrows [6]. The complete suppression of larval stages during development is only known for *Upogebia savignyi* (Strahl, 1862), a sponge commensal [91].

Species	Developmental stages	References
Callichirus major	ZI–ZV, M	[95]
Lepidophthalmus siriboia	Prezoea, ZI–ZIII, M, JI	[90]
Upogebia paraffinis	ZI–ZV, M	[89]
Upogebia vasquezi	ZI–ZIV, M	[48]

Note: Z, Zoea; M, Megalopa; J, juvenile. Roman numbers represent the number of developmental stages described.

Table 2. Thalassinidean species with occurrence on the coast of Pará whose larval and/or juvenile development stages have already been partially or completely described.

Thalassinideans have varying developmental patterns, generally one to eight zoeal stages [86, 92]. Among Axiidea, a reduced larval cycle is common, with two to three development stages (e.g., *Callichirus kraussi* (Stebbing, 1900) as *Callianassa kraussi* [93]; *Pestarella tyrrhena* (Petagna, 1792) as *C. tyrrhena* [22]; *Lepidophthalmus sinuensis* (Lemaitre and Rodrigues, 1991), *Lepidophthalmus louisianensis* (Schmitt, 1935) [94], and *L. siriboia* [90]). Some species in this group also have a long planktonic larval development, such as *C. major* and *Callichirus islagrande* (Schmitt, 1935), which undergo 4–5 zoeal stages [95, 96], or *Boasaxius princeps* (Boas, 1880) and *Nihonotrypaea petalura* (Stimpson, 1860), with 7–8 zoea [97, 98].

Regarding Gebiidea, a long larval development is frequent: *Naushonia crangonoides* (Kingsley, 1897) undergoes six to seven zoeal stages until it reaches the post-larval stage [99]; and *A. australis* (Rodrigues and Shimizu, 1992) shows up to eight zoeal stages [100]. The most common larval development pattern of *Upogebiidea* is the presence of three to four zoeal stages (e.g., *Upogebia kempi* (Shenoy, 1967) [101]; *Upogebia darwinii* (Miers, 1884) [102]; *U. major* [10]; *U. pusilla* [103]; *U. issaeffi* [104]; *U. yokoyai* [63]; *U. vasquezi* [48]).

The life cycle of *U. vasquezi* larvae has four zoeal stages [48]. When immature, the eggs of this species are yellowish (**Figure 5A**), their color start becoming more orange by the end of embryo development, in the hatching stage, when the eyes also become visible (**Figure 5B**). Larvae hatch in Zoea I, going through three other zoeal stages and one megalopa until reaching the first juvenile stage (**Figure 5C–H**).

Only *C. major*, *L. siriboia*, and *U. vasquezi* larvae have already been found in estuarine zooplankton samples from the Amazon coast [53]. Among the studies conducted with these species in the region, the taxonomic studies stand out, namely the morphological description of larval developmental stages of *L. siriboia* [90], as well as the description of mouth appendages and stomachs of larvae [105], analysis of the lecithotrophic behavior of this species during larval cycle [24], and abundance of larvae in the estuarine zooplankton [53]. With regard to *C. major*, the importance of feeding during larval development has been analyzed (as opposed to the lecithotrophic behavior of *L. siriboia*) [106], as well as the abundance of estuarine planktonic larvae throughout an annual cycle [53].

U. vasquezi was the most studied thalassinidean species in the region regarding larval biology, with description of larval morphology [48, 107], analysis of the effect of salinity on survival and duration of larval stages, its implication on larval migration [108], and occurrence of planktonic larvae along a salinity gradient in the Amazon estuary [53].

7.2. Effects of biotic factors on larval development

Diverse environmental factors influence developmental rates, number of stages, and survival of larvae of marine invertebrates [109]. Temperature and salinity are among the physicochemical factors that have a higher influence on survival and larval development of marine decapods [110]. Temperature might influence the growth of decapods during different life-cycle phases, from larvae and post-larvae to juveniles and adults [111], and trigger the acceleration or decrease of larval developmental rate, and impact metabolism and development, as well as

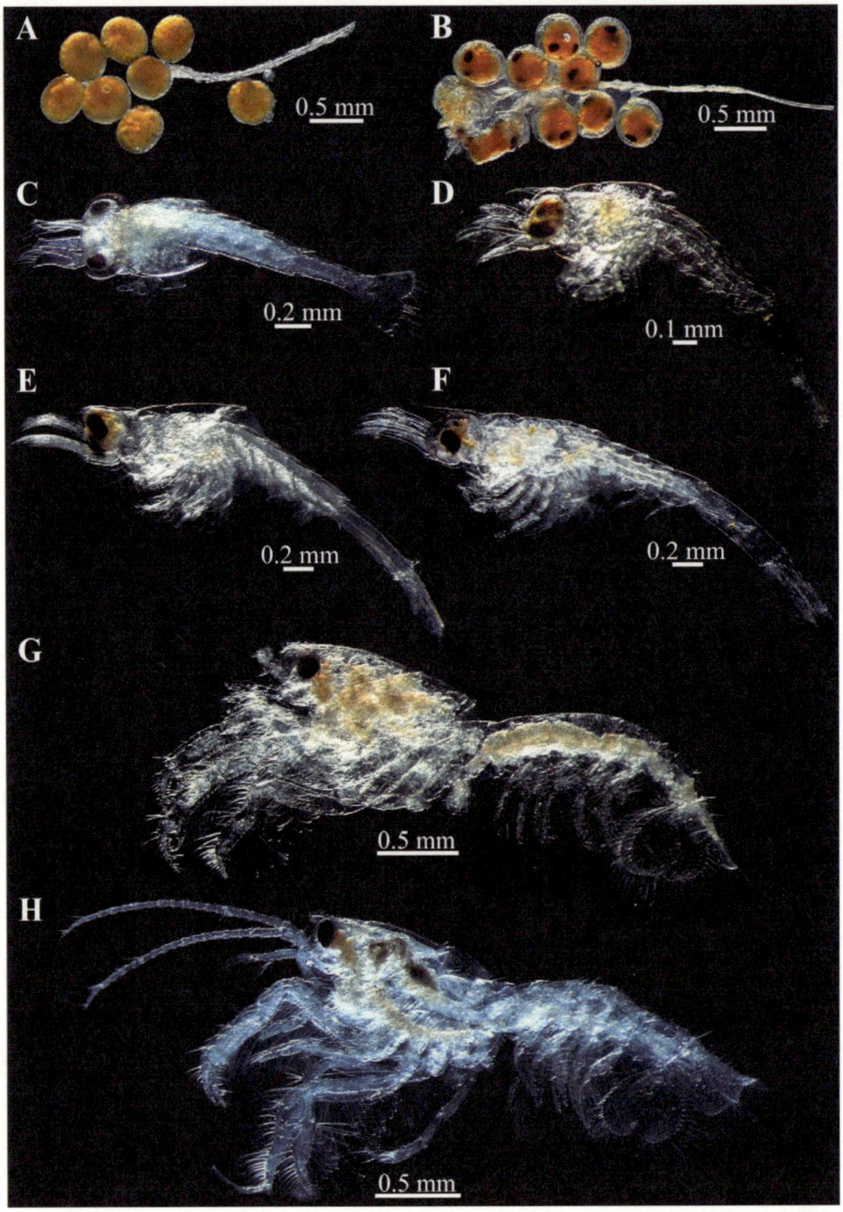

Figure 5. Developmental stages of *Upogebia vasquezi*. (A) Eggs in the initial developmental stage; (B) eggs in the final developmental stage; (C) Zoea I; (D) Zoea II; (E) Zoea III; (F) Zoea IV; (G) Megalopa (without antennas); (H) Juvenile I. Photos: Danielly Oliveira.

the seasonality of larvae emergence in some plankton species [110]. For instance, temperature mainly influences the duration of decapod larval stages, which are prolonged in stressful situations (for example, see [22, 112, 113]).

Saline concentration is generally constant in open sea, whereas it might seasonally fluctuate in coastal and estuarine zones, both regionally and locally [110]. Hence, salinity is considered an ecological and physiological factor of extreme importance for species in these environments [110], with impact on the development, survival, feeding, and growth rate, as well as on shedding cycles, metabolic rates, and behavior [113].

The reproductive behavior (life-cycle strategies) of decapods might also be influenced by salinity. Most estuarine species export their larvae to marine coastal zones, where salinity is more stable and, on average, higher than in the parental habitat, whereas others retain their initial larval stages inside the estuarine environment [112, 113]. For instance, some typical estuarine crabs increase their swimming activity in higher salinities to avoid being transported outside the estuary [114].

Studies analyzing the effect of salinity on larval development of decapods are also useful to identify which reproductive strategy is adopted by the species (either retention or exportation) due to the fact that saline limits tolerated by decapod larvae under experimental conditions coincide with their distribution along salinity gradients in the field [113]. In the coastal region of Pará, the effect of salinity on larval development of the crabs *Ucides cordatus* (Linnaeus, 1763), *Uca vocator* (Herbst, 1804), and *Uca rapax* was analyzed in the laboratory, obtaining decreased survival rates under lower salinity conditions, thus indicating a strategy of larval dispersal and exportation [115–118].

7.3. Reproduction, dynamics, and secondary production

Studies on the population dynamics and reproductive biology of thalassinideans have been developed in several locations worldwide, thus contributing to understanding the life cycle of these species (for example, see [14, 23, 80, 119–126]). Most of these studies were conducted in temperate and subtropical regions and few have shown estimates of population dynamic parameters for this group. On the Amazon coast, only the population dynamics of *L. siriboia* has been studied [59].

Secondary production might be defined as the production of biomass carried out by heterotrophic organisms, including animals, fungi, and heterotrophic bacteria; it represents an estimated biomass made available for higher trophic levels [127]. Decapod crustaceans have a crucial contribution to secondary production in the habitats they inhabit. For example, even though their abundance is lower than that of other invertebrates, they account for an important fraction of productivity in coral reef ecosystems [128] and on sandy beaches at different latitudes [129].

Secondary production estimates are still quite scarce, mostly in the equatorial region (between latitudes 5°S and 5°N), with absence of studies on benthic macrofaunal populations of sandy beaches [130]. Only 12 decapod populations have been studied [130] at higher latitudes, on tropical and subtropical beaches, including the thalassinids *U. pusilla* [4] and *C. major* [131, 132]. In Brazil, studies of this type have only been conducted in the Southern and Southeastern regions (for example, see [132–139]).

The capture of mud shrimps (Axiidea and Gebiidea) might cause changes in the target species and habitat and might influence resident communities and cause indirect effects on sediment structure [12, 13]). Excessive fishery efforts might lead to overexploitation of naturally abundant populations or even to the total disappearance of some species [12, 14]. Management plans and efforts for the conservation of these species and recovery of their habitats must be based on their regional population and reproductive characteristics [14]. Thus, studies that investigate population dynamics and reproductive biology of thalassinideans in several locations are of utmost importance, especially in priority conservation areas.

Despite the importance of thalassinidean species on Amazon coastal habitats, very little are known on their ecology, mostly regarding burrow morphology, physiology, population dynamics, behavior, and larval description.

Acknowledgements

The authors are grateful for the photos gently given by the colleagues: Dalila C. Silva (MSc) and Rory R. S. Oliveira (MSc). We also appreciate the valuable suggestions of the reviewers, which greatly improved the chapter. This study is part of the Ph.D. thesis of the first author (Danielly B. Oliveira) and was funded by the Brazilian National Research Council (CNPq) (Grant 553106/2005-8 to JMML), the Brazilian Higher Education Training Program (CAPES), and the Brazilian Carcinology Society (Grant SBC 01/2012). We also thank Daniela Tannus for translation of the original manuscript.

Author details

Danielly Brito de Oliveira[1,3]*, Fernando Araújo Abrunhosa[2] and Jussara Moretto Martinelli-Lemos[3]

*Address all correspondence to: danybrito@gmail.com

1 Center for Research and Management of Fishing Resources of the North Coast, Chico Mendes Institute for the Biodiversity Conservation (CEPNOR/ICMBIO), Belém, Pará, Brazil

2 Carcinology Laboratory, Federal University of Pará, Bragança, Pará, Brazil

3 Laboratory for Fishery Biology and Management of Aquatic Resources, Ecology of Amazonian Crustaceans Research Group (GPECA), Federal University of Pará, Belém, Pará, Brazil

References

[1] Rodrigues SA, Shimizu RM. Autoecologia de *Callichirus major* (Say, 1818). In: Absalão RS, Esteves AM, editors. Ecologia de praias arenosas do litoral brasileiro. Rio de Janeiro, UFRJ. Vol. III. Oecologia Brasiliensis. 1997. pp. 155-170

[2] Mclauhghlin PA, Camp DK, Angel MV, Bousfield EL, Brunei P, Brusca RC, Cadien D, Cohen AC, Conlan K, Eldredge LG, Felder DL, Goy JW, Haney T, Hann B, Heard RW,

Hendrycks A, Hobbs HH, Holsinger JR, Kensley B, Laubitz DR, Lecroy SE, Lemaitre R, Maddocks RF, Martin JW, Mikkelsen P, Nelson E, Newman WA, Overstreet RM, Poly WJ, Price WW, Reid JW, Robertson A, Rogers DC, Ross A, Schotte M, Schram FR, Shih C-T, Watling L, Wilson GDF. 2005. Common and scientific names of Aquatic Invertebrates from the United States and Canada: Crustaceans. Bethesda, Maryland: American Fisheries Society Special Publication 31. pp. 209-325

[3] Kornienko ES. Burrowing shrimp of the infraorders gebiidea and axiidea (Crustacea: Decapoda). Russian Journal of Marine Biology. 2013;**39**(1):1-14

[4] Dworschak PC. The biology of *Upogebia pusilla* (Petagna) (Decapoda, Thalassinidea). Growth and production. PSZNI Marine Ecology. 1988;**9**(1):51-77

[5] Coelho PA, Rattacaso MCA. Revisão das espécies de *Upogebia* encontradas em Pernambuco, Brasil (Crustacea, Decapoda, Thalassinidea). Revista Brasileira de Zoologia. 1988;**5**(3): 381-392. (Cessou em 2008. Cont. ISSN 1984-4670 Zoologia)

[6] Rodrigues SA, Pezzuto PR. Infraordem Thalassinidea (corruptos). In: Buckup L, Bond-Buckup G, editors. Os crustáceos do Rio Grande do Sul. Porto Alegre: Universidade/UFRGS; 1999. pp. 328-335

[7] Dworschak PC. Global diversity in the Thalassinidea (Decapoda). Journal of Crustacean Biology. 2000;**20**(2):238-245

[8] Ayón-Parente M, Hendrickx ME, Ríos-Jara E, Salgado-Barragán J. Records of mud shrimps (Crustacea: Decapoda: Axiidea and Gebiidae) from Pacific Mexico. Journal of the Marine Biological Association of the United Kingdom. 2014;**94**(2):369-388

[9] Silva DC, Martinelli-Lemos JM. Species composition and abundance of the benthic community of Axiidea and Gebiidea (Crustacea: Decapoda) in the Marapanim Bay, Amazon estuary, northern Brazil. Zoologia. 2012;**29**:144-158

[10] Konishi K. Larval development of the mud shrimp *Upogebia* (*Upogebia*) *major* (De Haan) (Crustacea: Thalassinidea: Upogebiidae) under laboratory conditions, with comments on larval characters of thalassinid families. Bulletin of National Research Institute of Aquaculture. 1989;**15**:1-17

[11] Hodgson AN, Allanson BR, Cretchley R. The exploitation of *Upogebia africana* (Crustacea: Thalassinidae) for bait in the Knysna Estuary. Transactions of the Royal Society of South Africa. 2000;**55**(2):197-204

[12] Souza JRB, Borzone CA. A extração de corrupto, *Callichirus major* (Say) (Crustacea, Thalassinidea), para uso como isca em praias do litoral do Paraná: As populações exploradas. Revista Brasileira de Zoologia. 2003;**20**(4):625-630. (Cessou em 2008. Cont. ISSN 1984-4670 Zoologia)

[13] Contessa L, Bird FL. The impact of bait-pumping on populations of the ghost shrimp *Trypaea australiensis* Dana (Decapoda: Callianassidae) and the sediment environment. Journal of Experimental Marine Biology and Ecology. 2004;**304**:75-97

[14] Botter-Carvalho ML, Santos PJP, Carvalho PVVC. Population dynamics of *Callichirus major* (Say, 1818) (Crustacea, Thalassinidea) on a beach in northeastern Brazil. Estuarine, Coastal and Shelf Science. 2007;**71**:508-516

[15] Conides AJ, Nicolaidou A, Apostolopoulou M, Thessalou-Legaki M. Growth, mortality and yield of the mudprawn *Upogebia pusilla* (Petagna, 1792) (Crustacea: Decapoda: Gebiidea) from western Greece. Acta Adriatica. 2012;**53**(1):87-103

[16] Brown AC, McLachlan A. Sandy shore ecosystems and the threats facing them: some predictions for the year 2025. Environmental Conservation. 2002;**29**(1):62-77

[17] Wynberg RP, Branch GM. Trampling associated with bait-collection for sandprawns *Callianassa kraussi* Stebbing: Effects on the biota of an intertidal sandflat. Environmental Conservation. 1997;**24**(2):139-148

[18] Shy JYA, Chan TY. Complete larval development of the edible mud shrimp *Upogebia edulis* Ngoc-Ho and Chan, 1992 (Decapoda: Thalassinidea: Upogebiidae) reared in the laboratory. Crustaceana. 1996;**69**(2):175-186

[19] Dumbauld BR, Armstrong DA, Feldman KL. Life-history characteristics of two sympatric thalassinidean shrimps, *Neotrypaea californiensis* and *Upogebia pugettensis*, with implications for oyster culture. Journal of Crustacean Biology. 1996;**16**(4):689-708

[20] Felder DL. Diversity and ecological significance of deep-burrowing macrocrustaceans in coastal tropical waters of the Americas (Decapoda: Thalassinidea). Interciencia. 2001;**26**(10):440-449

[21] Dumbauld BR, Wyllie-Echeverria S. The influence of burrowing thalassinid shrimps on the distribution of intertidal seagrasses in Willapa Bay, Washington, USA. Aquatic Botany. 2003;**77**:27-42

[22] Thessalou-Legaki M. Advanced larval development of *Callianassa tyrrhena* (Decapoda: Thalassinidea) and the effect of environmental factors. Journal of Crustacean Biology. 1990;**10**(4):659-666

[23] Candisani LC, Sumida PYG, Pires-Vanin AMS. Burrow morphology and mating behaviour of the thalassinidean shrimp *Upogebia noronhensis*. Journal of the Marine Biological Association of the United Kingdom. 2001;**81**(3795):1-5

[24] Abrunhosa FA, Simith DJB, Palmeira CAM, Arruda DCB. Lecithotrophic behaviour in zoea and megalopa larvae of the ghost shrimp *Lepidophthalmus siriboia* Felder and Rodrigues, 1993 (Decapoda: Callianassidae). Anais da Academia Brasileira de Ciências. 2008;**80**(4):639-646

[25] Coelho VR, Cooper RA, Rodrigues SA. Burrow morphology and behavior of the mud shrimp *Upogebia omissa* (Decapoda: Thalassinidea: Upogebiidae). Marine Ecology Progress Series. 2000;**200**:229-240

[26] Borradaile LA. On the classification of the Thalassinidea. Annals and Magazine of Natural History. 1903;**12**(7):534-551

[27] Hart JFL. Larval and adult stages of British Columbia Anomura. Canadian Journal of Research. 1937;**15**(10):179-220

[28] Mclauhghlin PA. Comparative Morphology of Recent Crustacea. San Francisco: W.H. Freeman and Company; 1980. p. 177

[29] Gurney R. Notes on some Decapod Crustacea from the Red Sea. VI–VIII. Proceedings of the Zoological Society of London. 1938;**108B**:73-84

[30] Gurney R. Larvae of Decapod Crustacea. London: Ray Society; 1942. p. 306

[31] Burkenroad MD. The higher taxonomy and evolution of Decapoda (Crustacea). Transactions of the San Diego Society of Natural History. 1981;**19**(17):251-268

[32] Poore GCB. A phylogeny of the families of Thalassinidea (Crustacea: Decapoda) with keys to families and genera. Memoirs of the Museum of Victoria. 1994;**54:**79-120

[33] Griffis RB, Suchanek TH. A model of burrow architecture and trophic modes in thalassinidean shrimp (Decapoda: Thalassinidea). Marine Ecology Progress Series. 1991;**79**:171-183

[34] Martin JW, Davis GE. An Updated Classification of the Recent Crustacea. Natural History Museum of Los Angeles Country. Los Angeles, California: Science Series; 2001;**39**:47-48

[35] Saint Laurent M. Sur la systématique et la phylogénie des Thalassinidea: définition des familles des Callianassidae et des Upogebiidae et diagnose de cinq genres nouveaux (Crustacea Decapoda). Comptes rendus hebdomadaires des séances de l'Académie des sciences, D. 1973;**277**:513-516

[36] Robles R, Tudge CC, Dworschak PC, Poore GCB, Felder DL. Molecular phylogeny of the Thalassinidea based on nuclear and mitochondrial genes. In: Martin JW, Crandall KA, Felder DL, editors. Crustacean Issues 18: Decapod Crustacean Phylogenetics. Boca Raton, FL: Taylor and Francis/CRC Press; 2009. pp. 309-326

[37] Lin FJ, Liu Y, Sha Z, Tsang LM, Chu KH, Chan TY, Liu R, Cui Z. Evolution and phylogeny of the mud shrimps (Crustacea: Decapoda) revealed from complete mitochondrial genomes. BMC Genomics. 2012;**13**:631-642

[38] De Grave S, Pentcheff ND, Ahyong ST, Chan TY, Crandall KA, Dworschak PC, Felder DL, Feldmann RM, Fransen CHJM, Goulding LYD, Lemaitre R, Low MEY, Martin JW, Ng PKL, Schweitzer CE, Tan SH, Tshudy D, Wetzer R. A classification of living and fossil genera of decapod crustaceans. Raffles Bulletin of Zoology. 2009;**21**:1-109

[39] Ahyong ST, Lowry JK, Alonso M, Bamber RN, Boxshall GA, Castro P, Gerken S, Karaman JS, Goy JW, Jones DS, Meland K, Rogers DC, Svavarsson J. subphylum crustacea brünnich, 1772. In: Zhang ZQ, editor. Animal Biodiversity: An Outline of Higher-level Classification and Survey of Taxonomic Richness. Zootaxa. 2011;**3148**:165-191

[40] Dworschak PC, Felder DL, Tudge CC. Infraorders Axiidea De Saint Laurent, 1979 and Gebiidea De Saint Laurent, 1979 (formerly known collectively as Thalassinidea). In:

Schran FR, Vaupel Klein JC, editors. The Crustacea – Treatise on Zoology: Anatomy, Taxonomy, Biology. Boston: Koninklijke Brill NV; 2012. Crustacea. 9B(69). pp. 109-219

[41] Dworschak PC. Axiidea and Gebiidea (Crustacea: Decapoda) of Costa Rica. Annalen des Naturhistorischen Museums in Wien. 2013;**115**(B):37-55

[42] Poore GCB, Ahyong ST, Bracken-Grissom HD, Chan TY, Chu KH, Crandall KA, Dworschak PC, Felder DL, Feldmann RM, Hyžný M, Karasawa H, Lemaitre R, Komai T, Li X, Mantelatto FL, Martin JW, Ngoc-Ho N, Robles R, Schweitzer CE, Tamaki A, Tsang LM, Tudge CC. On stabilising the names of the infraorders of thalassinidean shrimps, Axiidea de Saint Laurent, 1979 and Gebiidea de Saint Laurent, 1979 (Decapoda). Crustaceana. 2014;**87**:1258-1272

[43] Sakai K, Turkay M. A review of the collections of the Infraorders Thalassinidea Latreille, 1831 and Callianassidea Dana, 1852 (Decapoda, Pleocyemata) lodged in three German museums, with revised keys to the genera and species. Crustaceana. 2014;**87**(2):129-211

[44] Saint Laurent M. Vers une nouvelle classification des Crustacés Décapodes Reptantia. Bulletin de l'Office National des Pêches République Tunisienne. 1979;**3**:15-31

[45] Dworschak PC. Methods collecting Axiidea and Gebiidea (Decapoda): A review. Annalen des Naturhistorischen Museums in Wien. 2015;**117**(B):5-21

[46] Wear RG, Yaldwyn JC. Studies on Thalassinid Crustacea (Decapoda, Macrura Reptantia) with a Description of a New Jaxea from New Zelan and an Account of its Larval Development. Vol. 41. Zoology Publications from Victoria University of Wellington, New Zealand; 1966

[47] Melo GAS. Manual de identificação dos Crustacea Decapoda do litoral brasileiro: Anomura, Thalassinidea, Palinuridea e Astacidea. São Paulo: Plêiade/FAPESP; 1999. p. 551

[48] Oliveira DB, Martinelli-Lemos JM, Abrunhosa FA. The complete larval development of the mud shrimp *Upogebia vasquezi* (Gebiidea: Upogebiidae) reared in the laboratory. Zootaxa. 2014;**3826**(3):517-543

[49] Dworschak PC. Global diversity in the Thalassinidea (Decapoda): An update (1998-2004). Nauplius. 2005;**13**(1):57-63

[50] Sakai K. Upogebiidae of the world. Crustacean Monographs. 2006;**6**:1-185

[51] Nucci PR, Melo GAS. First record of *Upogebia inomissa* Williams, 1993 (Decapoda, Thalassinidea, Upogebiidae) in Brazil. Nauplius. 2001;**9**(1):71-71

[52] Barros MP, Pimentel FR. A fauna de Decapoda (Crustacea) do Estado do Pará, Brasil: lista preliminar das espécies. Boletim do Museu Paraense Emílio Goeldi, Zoologia. 2001;**17**(1):15-41

[53] Oliveira DB, Silva DC, Martinelli JM. Density of larval and adult forms of the burrowing crustaceans *Lepidophthalmus siriboia* (Callianassidae) and *Upogebia vasquezi* (Upogebiidae) in an Amazon estuary, northern Brazil. Journal of the Marine Biological Association of the United Kingdom. 2012;**92**(2):295-303

[54] Hernández-Ávila I, Lira C, Hernández G, Bolaños J. *Upogebia vasquezi* Ngoc-Ho, 1989 (Decapoda: Thalassinidea: Upogebiidae): First record for Venezuela. Boletin del Instituto Oceanografico de Venezuela. 2005;**44**(2):119-122

[55] Souza Filho PWM. Costa de manguezais de macromaré da Amazônia: cenários morfológicos, mapeamento e quantificação de áreas usando dados de sensores remotos. Revista Brasileira de Geofísica. 2005;**23**(4):427-435

[56] Burke L, Kura Y, Kassem K, Revenga C, Spalding M, Mcallister D. Coastal Ecosystems. Washington: World Resources Institute; 2001. disponível em: http://www.wri.org/wr2000. (Acesso em fevereiro de 2015)

[57] Vilhena MPSP, Costa ML, Berrêdo JF. Continental and marine contributions to formation of mangrove sediments in an Eastern Amazonian mudplain: The case of the Marapanim Estuary. Journal of South American Earth Sciences. 2010;**29**:427-438

[58] Silva CA, Souza-Filho PW, Rodrigues SWP. Morphology and modern sedimentary deposits of the macrotidal Marapanim Estuary (Amazon, Brazil). Continental Shelf Research. 2008;**29**:619-631

[59] Rosa-Filho JS, Girard TC, Frédou FL. Population dynamics of the burrowing shrimp *Lepidophthalmus siriboia* Felder and Rodrigues, 1993 (Reptantia: Axiidea: Callianassidae) on the Amazonian coast. Journal of Crustacean Biology. 2013;**33**(4):503-511

[60] Laverock B, Smith CJ, Tait K, Osborn AM, Widdicombe S, Gilbert JA. Bioturbating shrimp alter the structure and diversity of bacterial communities in coastal marine sediments. The International Society for Microbial Ecology Journal. 2010;**4**:1531-1544

[61] Laverock B, Kitidis V, Tait K, Gilbert JA, Osborn AM, Widdicombe S. Bioturbation determines the response of benthic ammonia-oxidizing microorganisms to ocean acidification. Philosophical Transactions of The Royal Society, Biological Sciences. 2013;**368**:20120441. Available from: http://dx.doi.org/10.1098/rstb.2012.0441

[62] Laverock B, Tait K, Gilbert JA, Osborn AM, Widdicombe S. Impacts of bioturbation on temporal variation in bacterial and archaeal nitrogen-cycling gene abundance in coastal sediments. Environmental Microbiology Reports. 2014;**6**(1):113-121

[63] Kornienko ES, Korn OM, Demchuk DD. The larval development of the mud shrimp *Upogebia yokoyai* Makarov, 1938 (Decapoda: Gebiidea: Upogebiidae) reared under laboratory conditions. Journal of Natural History. 2013;**47**(29-30):1933-1952

[64] Sasaki A, Nakao H, Yoshitake S, Nakatsubo T. Effects of the burrowing mud shrimp, *Upogebia yokoyai*, on carbon flow and microbial activity on a tidal flat. Ecological Research. 2014;**29**:493-499

[65] Webb AP, Eyre BD. Effect of natural populations of burrowing thalassinidean shrimp on sediment irrigation, benthic metabolism, nutrient fluxes and denitrification. Marine Ecology Progress Series. 2004;**268**:205-220

[66] Kinoshita K. Burrow structure of the mud shrimp *Upogebia major* (Decapoda: Thalassinidea: Upogebiidae). Journal of Crustacean Biology. 2002;**22**(2):474-480

[67] Berkenbusch K, Rowden AA. An examination of the spatial and temporal generality of the influence of ecosystem engineers on the composition of associated assemblages. Aquatic Ecology. 2007;**41**:129-147

[68] Hernáez P, Wehrtmann IS. Population of the burrowing shrimp *Callichirus seilacheri* (Decapoda: Callianassidae) in northern Chile. Revista de Biología Tropical. 2007;**55**:141-152

[69] Allanson BR, Skinner D, Imberger J. Flow in prawn burrows. Estuarine, Coastal and Shelf Science. 1992;**35**:253-266

[70] Astall CM, Taylor AC, Atkinson RJA. Behavioural and physiological implications of a burrow-dwelling lifestyle for two species of Upogebiid mud-shrimp (Crustacea: Thalassinidea). Estuarine, Coastal and Shelf Science. 1997;**44**:155-168

[71] Atkinson RJA, Froglia C, Arneri E, Antolini B. Observations on the burrows and burrowing behavior of *Brachynotus gemmellari* and on the burrows of several other species occurring on *Squilla* grounds off Ancona, Central Adriatic. Scientia Marina. 1998;**62**(1-2):91-100

[72] Curran HA, Martin AJ. Complex decapod burrows and ecological relationships in modern and Pleistocene intertidal carbonate environments, San Salvador Island, Bahamas. Palaeogeography, Palaeoclimatology, Palaeoecology. 2003;**192**:229-245

[73] Sepahvand V, Sari A, Tudge C, Bolouki M. A study of burrow morphology in representative axiidean and gebiidean mud shrimps, from the Persian Gulf and Gulf of Oman, Iran. Nauplius. 2014;**22**(2):137-144

[74] Kinoshita K, Itani G, Uchino T. Burrow morphology and associated animals of the mud shrimp *Upogebia yokoyai* (Crustacea: Thalassinidea: Upogebiidae). Journal of the Marine Biological Association of the United Kingdom. 2010;**90**(5):947-952

[75] Macginite GE. The natural history of *Callianassa californiensis* Dana. American Midland Naturalist. 1934;**15**(2):166-177

[76] Santagata S. A waterborne behavioral cue for the actinotroch larva of *Phoronis pallida* (Phoronida) produced by *Upogebia pugettensis* (Decapoda: Thalassinidea). Biological Bulletin. 2004;**207**:103-115

[77] Lima JF, Abrunhosa F, Coelho PA. The larval development of *Pinnixa gracilipes* Coelho (Decapoda, Pinnotheridae) reared in the laboratory. Revista Brasileira de Zoologia. 2006;**23**(2):480-489

[78] Anker A, Jeng MS, Chan TY. Two unusual species of Alpheidae (Decapoda: Caridea) associated with upogebiid mud shrimps in the mudflats of Taiwan and Vietnam. Journal of Crustacean Biology. 2001;**21**(4):1048-1061

[79] Peiró DF, Baeza JA, Mantelatto FL. Host-use pattern and sexual dimorphism reveals the mating system of the symbiotic pea crab *Austinixa aidae* (Crustacea: Brachyura: Pinnotheridae). Journal of the Marine Biological Association of the United Kingdom. 2013;**93**:715-723

[80] Botter-Carvalho ML, Costa LB, Gomes LL, Clemente CCC, Carvalho PVVC. Reproductive biology and population structure of *Axianassa australis* (Crustacea, Axianassidae) on a sand-mud flat in north-eastern Brazil. Journal of the Marine Biological Association of the United Kingdom. 2015;**95**(4):735-745

[81] Dumbauld BR, Chapman JW, Torchin ME, Kuris AM. Is the collapse of mud shrimp (*Upogebia pugettensis*) populations along the Pacific Coast of North America caused by outbreaks of a previously unknown bopyrid isopod parasit (*Orthione griffenis*)? Estuaries and Coasts. 2011;**34**:336-350

[82] Chapman JW, Dumbauld BR, Itani G, Markham JC. An introduced Asian parasite threatens northeastern Pacific estuarine ecosystems. Biological Invasions. 2012;**14**:1221-1236

[83] Ubaldo JP, Nanri T, Takada Y, Saigusa M. Prevalence and patterns of infection by the epicaridean parasite, *Gyge ovalis* and the emergence of intersex in the estuarine mud shrimp, *Upogebia major*. Journal of the Marine Biological Association of the United Kingdom. 2014;**94**(3):557-566

[84] Selin NI. Some features of the biology of the mud shrimp *Upogebia issaeffi* (Balls, 1913) (Decapoda: Upogebiidae) from the Subtidal Zone of Vostok Bay, Sea of Japan. Russian Journal of Marine Biology. 2014;**40**(1):24-29

[85] Henmi Y, Itani G. Burrow utilization in the goby *Eutaeniichthys gilli* associated with the Mud shrimp *Upogebia yokoyai*. Zoological Science. 2014;**31**(8):523-528

[86] Pohle G, Santana W. Gebiidea and axiidea (= thalassinidea). In: Martin JW, Olesen J, Høeg JT, editors. Atlas of Crustacean Larvae. Baltimore, MD: Johns Hopkins University Press; 2014

[87] Pohle G, Santana W, Jansen G, Greenlaw M. Plankton-caught zoeal stages and megalopa of the lobster shrimp *Axius serratus* (Decapoda: Axiidae) from the Bay of Fundy, Canada, with a summary of axiidean and gebiidean literature on larval descriptions. Journal of Crustacean Biology. 2011;**31**(1):82-99

[88] Andryszak BL. *Upogebia affinis* (Say): Its postlarval stage described from Louisiana plankton, with a comparison to postlarvae of other species within the genus and notes on its distribution. Journal of Crustacean Biology. 1986;**6**(2):214-226

[89] Melo SG, Brossi-Garcia AL. Postembryonic development of *Upogebia paraffinis* Williams, 1993 (Decapoda, Thalassinidea), reared under laboratory conditions. Nauplius. 2000;**8**(1):149-168

[90] Abrunhosa FA, Pires MAB, Lima JF, Coelho-Filho PA. Larval development of *Lepidophthalmus siriboia* Felder and Rodrigues, 1993 (Thalassinidea) from the Amazon region, reared in the laboratory. Acta Amazonica. 2005;**35**(1):77-84

[91] Gurney R. Notes on some Decapod Crustacea from the Red Sea. II. The larvae of *Upogebia savignyi* (Strahl). Proceedings of the Zoological Society of London. 1937;**107**B:85-101

[92] Rabalais NN, Gore RH. Abbreviated development in decapods. In: Wenner AM, editor. Crustacean Growth: Larval Growth. (Gen. Ed. Frederik R. Schram, San Diego). Crustacean Issues. 1985;**2**:67-126. ISBN 9061912946

[93] Forbes AT. An unusual abbreviated larval life in the estuarine burrowing prawn *Callianassa kraussi* (Crustacea: Decapoda: Thalassinidea). Marine Biology. Springer Berlin Heidelberg; 1973;**22**:361-365

[94] Nates SF, Felder DL, Lemaitre R. Comparative larval development in two species of the burrowing ghost shrimp genus *Lepidophthalmus* (Decapoda: Callianassidae). Journal of Crustacean Biology. 1997;**17**(3):497-519

[95] Strasser KM, Felder DL. Larval development in two populations of the ghost shrimp *Callichirus major* (Decapoda: Thalassinidea) under laboratory conditions. Journal of Crustacean Biology. 1999;**19**(4):844-878

[96] Strasser KL, Felder DL. Larval development of the ghost shrimp *Callichirus islagrande* (Decapoda: Thalassinidea: Callianassidae) under laboratory conditions. Journal of Crustacean Biology. 2000;**20**(1):100-117

[97] Kornienko ES, Korn OM, Golubinskaya DD. The complete larval development of the lobster shrimp *Boasaxius princeps* Boas, 1880 (Decapoda: Axiidea: Axiidae) obtained in the laboratory. Journal of Natural History. 2014;**48**(29-30):1737-1769

[98] Kornienko ES, Korn OM, Golubinskaya DD. The number of zoeal stages in larval development of *Nihonotrypaea petalura* (Stimpson, 1860) (Decapoda: Axiidea: Callianassidae) from Russian waters of the Sea of Japan. Zootaxa. 2015;**3919**(2):343-361

[99] Goy JW, Provenzano Jr. AJ. Larval development of the rare burrowing mud shrimp *Naushonia crangonoides* Kingsley (Decapoda: Thalassinidea; Laomediidae). Biological Bulletin. 1978;**154**(2):241-261

[100] Strasser KM, Felder DL. Larval development of the mud shrimp *Axianassa australis* (Decapoda: Thalassinidea) under laboratory conditions. Journal of Natural History. 2005;**39**(25):2289-2306

[101] Shenoy S. Studies on larval development in Anomura (Crustacea, Decapoda) – II. Proceedings of the Symposium on Crustacea, II. Mandapam Camp: Marine Biological Association of India. 1967. p. 777-804

[102] Ngoc-Ho N. The larval development of Upogebia darwini (Crustacea, Thalassinidea) reared in the laboratory, with a redescription of the adult. Proceeding of the Zoological Society of London. 1977;**181**:439-464

[103] Santos A, Paula J. Redescription of the larval stages of *Upogebia pusilla* (Petagna, 1792) (Thalassinidea, Upogebiidae) from laboratory-reared material. Invertebrate Reproduction and Development. 2003;**43**(1):83-90

[104] Kornienko ES, Korn OM, Demchuk DD. The larval development of the mud shrimp *Upogebia issaeffi* (Balss, 1913) (Decapoda: Gebiidea: Upogebiidae) reared under laboratory conditions. Zootaxa. 2012;**3269**:31-46

[105] Abrunhosa FA, Melo M, Lima JF, Abrunhosa J. Developmental morphology of mouthparts and foregut of the larvae and postlarvae of *Lepidophthalmus siriboia* Felder and Rodrigues, 1993 (Decapoda: Callianassidae). Acta Amazonica. 2006;**36**(3):335-342

[106] Abrunhosa FA, Arruda DCB, Simith DJB, Palmeira CAM. The importance of feeding in the larval development of the ghost shrimp *Callichirus major* (Decapoda: Callianassidae). Anais da Academia Brasileira de Ciências. 2008;**80**(3):445-453

[107] Oliveira DB, Martinelli JM, Abrunhosa FA. Description of early larval stages of *Upogebia vasquezi* (Gebiidea: Upogebiidae) reared in laboratory. Journal of the Marine Biological Association of the United Kingdom. 2012;**92**(2):335-342

[108] Oliveira DB, Martinelli-Lemos JM, Souza AS, Costa JR, Abrunhosa FA. Does retention or exportation occur in the larvae of the mud shrimp *Upogebia vasquezi* (Decapoda, Gebiidea)? Implications for the reproductive strategy of the species on the Amazon coast. Hydrobiologia. 2016;**773**:241-252

[109] Costlow JD, Bookhout CG, Monroe R. The effect of salinity and temperature on larval development of *Sesarma cinereum* (Bosc) reared in the laboratory. Biological Bulletin. 1960;**118**(2):183-202

[110] Anger K. The Biology of Decapod Crustacean Larvae. Crustacean Issues, Zoological Museum. University of Amsterdam, CRC Press; 2001. pp. 1-300

[111] Hartnoll RG. Growth in Crustacea – twenty years on. In: Paula JPM, Flores AAV, Fransen CHJM, editors. Advances in Decapod Crustacean Research. Hydrobiologia. Kluwer Academic Publishers, Netherlands; 2001;**449**:111-122

[112] Paula J, Mendes RN, Paci S, Mclaughlin P, Gherardi F, Emmerson W. Combined effects of temperature and salinity on the larval development of the estuarine mud prawn *Upogebia africana* (Crustacea, Thalassinidea). Hydrobiologia. 2001;**449**:141-148

[113] Anger K. Salinity as a key parameter in the larval biology of decapod crustaceans. Invertebrate Reproduction and Development. 2003;**43**(1):29-45

[114] Queiroga H, Blanton J. Interactions between behaviour and physical forcing in the control of horizontal transport of decapod crustacean larvae. Advances in Marine Biology. 2005;**47**:107-214

[115] Diele K, Simith DJB. Salinity tolerance of northern Brazilian mangrove crab larvae, *Ucides cordatus* (Ocypodidae): Necessity for larval export? Estuarine, Coastal and Shelf Science. 2006;**68**:600-608

[116] Simith DJB, Diele K. O efeito da salinidade no desenvolvimento larval do caranguejo - uçá, *Ucides cordatus* (Linnaeus, 1763) (Decapoda: Ocypodidae) no Norte do Brasil. Acta Amazonica. 2008;**38**(2):345-350

[117] Simith DJB, Souza AS, Maciel CR, Abrunhosa FA, Diele K. Influence of salinity on the larval development of the fiddler crab *Uca vocator* (Ocypodidae) as an indicator of ontogenetic migration towards offshore waters. Helgolang Marine Research. 2012;**66**:77-85

[118] Simith DJB, Pires MAB, Abrunhosa FA, Maciel CR, Diele K. Is larval dispersal a necessity for decapod crabs from the Amazon mangroves? Response of *Uca rapax* zoeae to different salinities and comparison with sympatric species. Journal of Experimental Marine Biology and Ecology. 2014;**457**:22-30

[119] Tamaki A, Ingole B. Distribution of juvenile and adult ghost shrimps, *Callianassa japonica* Ortmann (Thalassinidea), on an intertidal sand flat: Intraspecific facilitation as a possible pattern-generating factor. Journal of Crustacean Biology. 1993;**13**(1):175-183

[120] Kevrekidis T, Gouvis N, Koukouras A. Population dynamics, reproduction and growth of *Upogebia pusilla* (Decapoda, Thalassinidea) in the Evros Delta (North Aegean Sea). Crustaceana. 1997;**70**(7):799-812

[121] Pezzuto PR. Population dynamics of *Sergio mirim* (Rodrigues 1971) (Decapoda: Thalassinidea: Callianassidae) in Cassino Beach, southern Brazil. Marine Ecology – Pubblicazioni del la Stazione Zoologica di Napoli I. 1998;**19**:89-109

[122] Nates SF, Felder DL. Growth and maturation of the ghost shrimp *Lepidophthalmus sinuensis* Lemaitre and Rodrigues, 1991 (Crustacea, Decapoda, Callianassidae), a burrowing pest in penaeid shrimp culture ponds. Fishery Bulletin. 1999;**97**:526-541

[123] Berkenbusch K, Rowden AA. Latitudinal variation in the reproductive biology of the burrowing ghost shrimp *Callianassa filholi* (Decapoda: Thalassinidea). Marine Biology. 2000;**136**:497-504

[124] Tamaki A, Miyabe S. Larval abundance patterns for three species of *Nihonotrypaea* (Decapoda: Thalassinidea: Callianassidae) along an estuary-to-open-sea gradient in Western Kyushu, Japan. Journal of Crustacean Biology. 2000;**20**(2):182-191

[125] Kinoshita K, Nakayama S, Furota T. Life cycle characteristics of the deep-burrowing mud shrimp *Upogebia major* (Thalassinidea: Upogebiidae) on a tidal flat along the northern coast of Tokyo bay. Journal of Crustacean Biology. 2003;**23**(2):318-327

[126] Rotherham D, West RJ. Patterns in reproductive dynamics of burrowing ghost shrimp *Trypaea australiensis* from small to intermediate scales. Marine Biology. 2009;**156**:1277-1287

[127] Kaiser MJ, Attrill MJ, Jennings S, Thomas DN, Barnes DKA, Brierley AS, Hiddink JG, Kaartokallio H, Polunin NVC, Raffaelli DG. Marine Ecology: Processes, Systems, and Impacts. 2nd ed. Oxford: OUP; 2011. p. 528

[128] Kramer MJ, Bellwood DR, Bellwood O. Benthic Crustacea on coral reefs: A quantitative survey. Marine Ecology Progress Series. 2014;**511**:105-116

[129] Petracco M, Cardoso RS, Corbisier TN, Turra A. Brazilian sandy beach macrofauna production: A review. Brazilian Journal of Oceanography. 2012;**60**(4):473-484

[130] Petracco M, Cardoso RS, Turra A. Patterns of sandy-beach macrofauna production. Journal of the Marine Biological Association of the United Kingdom. 2013;**93**(7):1717-1725

[131] Souza JRB, Borzone CA, Brey T. Population dynamics and secondary production of *Callichirus major* (Crustacea: Thalassinidea) on a southern Brazilian sandy beach. Archives of Fisheries and Marine Research. 1998;**46**:151-164

[132] Petracco M. Produção secundária da macrofauna bentônica da zona entremarés no segmento norte da praia do Uma, litoral sul do estado de São Paulo [Phd Thesis]. São Paulo: University of São Paulo; 2008. p. 254

[133] Cardoso RS, Veloso VG. Population biology and secondary production of the sand-hopper *Pseudorchestoidea brasiliensis* (Amphipoda: Talitridae) at Prainha Beach, Brazil. Marine Ecology Progress Series. 1996;**142**:111-119

[134] Petracco M, Veloso VG, Cardoso RS. Population dynamics and secondary production of *Emerita brasiliensis* (Crustacea: Hippidae) at Prainha Beach, Brazil. Marine Ecology. 2003;**24**(3):231-245

[135] Veloso VG, Cardoso RS, Petracco M. Secondary production of the intertidal Macrofauna of Prainha Beach, Brazil. Journal of Coast Research. 2003;**35**:385-391

[136] Souza JRB, Borzone CA. Population dynamics and secondary production of *Euzonus furciferus* Ehlers (Polychaeta, Opheliidae) in an exposed sandy beach of Southern Brazil. Revista Brasileira de Zoologia. 2007;**24**(4):1139-1144

[137] Veloso VG, Sallorenzo IA. Differences in the secondary production of *Emerita brasiliensis* (Decapoda: Hippidae) on two sandy beaches in Rio de Janeiro State, Brazil. Nauplius. 2010;**18**(1):57-68

[138] Petracco M, Cardoso RS, Corbisier TN, Turra A. Secondary production of sandy beach macrofauna: An evaluation of predictive models. Estuarine, Coastal and Shelf Science. 2012;**115**:359-365

[139] Turra A, Petracco M, Amaral AC, Denadai MR. Population biology and secondary production of the harvested clam *Tivela mactroides* (Born, 1778) (Bivalvia, Veneridae) in Southeastern Brazil. Marine Ecology. 2015;**36**(2):221-234